# I GOT THIS

# JENNIFER HUDSON

# I GOT THIS

*How I Changed My Ways and*

*Lost What Weighed Me Down*

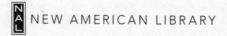
NEW AMERICAN LIBRARY

NEW AMERICAN LIBRARY
Published by New American Library, a division of
Penguin Gro up (USA) Inc., 375 Hudson Street,
New York, New York 10014, USA
Penguin Group (Canada), 90 Eglinton Avenue East, Suite 700, Toronto,
Ontario M4P 2Y3, Canada (a division of Pearson Penguin Canada Inc.)
Penguin Books Ltd., 80 Strand, London WC2R 0RL, England
Penguin Ireland, 25 St. Stephen's Green, Dublin 2,
Ireland (a division of Penguin Books Ltd.)
Penguin Group (Australia), 250 Camberwell Road, Camberwell, Victoria 3124,
Australia (a division of Pearson Australia Group Pty. Ltd.)
Penguin Books India Pvt. Ltd., 11 Community Centre, Panchsheel Park,
New Delhi - 110 017, India
Penguin Group (NZ), 67 Apollo Drive, Rosedale, Auckland 0632,
New Zealand (a division of Pearson New Zealand Ltd.)
Penguin Books (South Africa) (Pty.) Ltd., 24 Sturdee Avenue,
Rosebank, Johannesburg 2196, South Africa

Penguin Books Ltd., Registered Offices:
80 Strand, London WC2R 0RL, England

Published by New American Library, a division of Penguin Group (USA) Inc. Previously published in a Dutton hardcover edition.

First New American Library Printing, January 2013
10   9   8   7   6   5   4   3   2

 REGISTERED TRADEMARK—MARCA REGISTRADA

New American Library Trade Paperback ISBN: 978-0-451-23912-9

The Library of Congress has cataloged the hardcover edition of this title as follows:

Hudson, Jennifer, 1981–
    I got this: how I changed my ways and lost what weighed me down/Jennifer Hudson.
        p. cm.
    ISBN 978-0-525-95277-0
    1. Hudson, Jennifer, 1981–. 2. Singers—United States—Biography. 3. Motion picture actors and actresses—United States—Biography. 4. Overweight persons—United States—Biography. I. Title.
    ML420.H835A3 2012
    782.42164092—dc23
    [B]

Printed in the United States of America

Set in Walbaum MT Std
Designed by Alissa Amell

PUBLISHER'S NOTE
Penguin is committed to publishing works of quality and integrity. In that spirit, we are proud to offer this book to our readers; however the story, the experiences and the words are the author's alone.

The recipes contained in this book are to be followed exactly as written. The publisher is not responsible for your specific health or allergy needs that may require medical supervision. The publisher is not responsible for any adverse reactions to the recipes contained in this book.

Accordingly nothing in this book is intended as an express or implied warranty of the suitability or fitness of any product, service or design. The reader wishing to use a product, service or design discussed in this book should first consult a specialist or professional to ensure suitability and fitness for the reader's particular lifestyle and environmental needs.

*To my cousin Angela White—who is the ultimate health*

*fanatic, my workout buddy, and a huge part of my inspiration.*

# CONTENTS

# I GOT THIS

# INTRODUCTION

"**J**ennifer! Over here!"

"Jennifer, look this way."

"Jennifer, Jennifer."

"Over here!"

"No, over here!"

"Jennifer, turn to the right!"

I always dreamed of someday walking the red carpet in Hollywood. Let's be real. It's fun. Everyone there is shouting out your name just to get a glimpse of what you're wearing. The press asks you to pose, wave, and smile as they snap photo after photo, with flashes popping so bright you can hardly see. It's a moment in time a girl feels truly beautiful. And on this particular night, I thought I was looking fierce.

It was one of my first red-carpet events. I was a contestant on *American Idol*, and was living my dream of singing for millions of people on the highest-rated show on television. I was a long way from singing in church and talent shows on the South Side of

Chicago. I was excited, taking in the red-carpet finery for the first time. I felt on top of the world.

"Jennifer, are you insecure about being a 'big girl' in Hollywood?"

That is, until *that* question.

Oh, *hell* no. She didn't just ask me that.

But she did.

It took me a minute to figure out who the reporter was actually talking to.

Who, me? I thought. Insecure?

Surely, she wasn't addressing *me* that way. I had the height of a supermodel, breasts that were naturally big *and* real, and a God-given shape. Why would I feel insecure about that? I looked around hoping to spot another Jennifer—an insecure "big" girl, but there wasn't anyone else there.

Nope.

Just me.

Like Randy Jackson said to me after my *American Idol* audition: "Welcome to Hollywood, girl!"

# CHAPTER ONE

## BELIEVE

I was born on September 12, 1981, in the Englewood area of Chicago. I am the third child of my parents, Darnell Hudson Donnerson and Samuel Simpson. My mama raised me, my sister, Julia, and my brother, Jason on her own as a single parent. We were a close family, surrounded by lots of aunts, uncles, cousins, and our grandparents.

I come from the South Side of Chicago, where a lot of the girls have curves. Most of the men there don't want their ladies too skinny. Oh, no. They want a little meat on the bones, and a little something to hold on to. Most of the girls in my neighborhood were built just like me—and that's what we wanted. Now, I don't know about you, but I'd much rather have my share of nice curves than no shape at all. That's not to say that I didn't know I was bigger than some girls—I just never really felt all that insecure about it.

My sister, Julia, has been a big girl for her entire life. My brother, Jason, was built exactly the same.

As for me?

Comparatively speaking, I was the skinny one in my family! In fact, I was so thin as a little girl that you could see my ribs beneath my shirts. My mama took me, not Julia and Jason—the heavy kids in our family—to the doctor. She thought something had to be wrong.

"My child must be very sick! I can see her ribs!" Mama spoke desperately to the doctor as if I was dying. I wasn't sick and I surely wasn't dying—I was just *thin*.

In my family, if you were too skinny, something *had* to be wrong. My family likes to see some shape, too, and if you don't have that, they'll feed you until you do. And trust me—when it comes to food, the Hudsons don't play around.

Like a lot of families in my neighborhood, food was a central focus for all types of gatherings, from family reunions to Sunday-night dinners. There were, of course, the exceptions, and I grew up knowing kids from school who were rarely served home-cooked meals—they ate TV dinners and frozen vegetables—but that wasn't our family. My mama would never allow that kind of food in our house. She loved to cook. I never knew times were tough or that money was short in our home because Mama always had a hot meal on the table. And if she cooked it, we ate it. My grandma and mama were the best cooks, and later, Jason became a good cook, too. Not me—I didn't start cooking much until I got older and had a family of my own.

It gave my mama a lot of joy to make meals for her kids. She especially loved making hot breakfasts so we could start our days off right and nourished. Before school, we filled our plates with bacon, ham or sausage, pancakes, waffles, eggs, and biscuits. I said *nourished* . . . not healthy! But oh, that food was so good.

When it came time for dinner, meals were always prepared fresh and from scratch, too. We were a family of tradition and creatures of habit, so Wednesday was spaghetti night, Friday was always our fried fish night, and Sunday was strictly about praising God, spending time with family, and eating really good food. We'd all go to church in the morning and then stop someplace after service for a bite to eat for lunch. Sundays were the only day of the week that we ate out. It was a special treat I looked forward to every week. My grandma and mama loved to stop at Kentucky Fried Chicken, but we kids always wanted to eat at McDonald's. I usually ordered a cheeseburger with *no* onions—I hated onions as a kid and still do. If my burger came with onions, I'd sit there, cry, and refuse to eat it until my mama picked the onions off—or my brother ate my burger for me.

Whenever we ate out, I nitpicked my meal so I could make it last longer, and I was a slow eater, anyway. Eating out was that much of a treat. We weren't allowed to order a drink because it cost too much money. Mind you, this was before the days of value meals, so everything on the menu was à la carte. Jason told my mama that if he didn't have a drink, he'd throw up his food. That was his way of being slick to get himself a drink. It worked every time, too.

Sunday nights were full-on family-style dinners with all the fixings. Those meals were like a traditional Christmas dinner at my mama's house every week, with most of my favorite foods being served—collard greens, creamy mashed potatoes, pork chops with heavy gravy, macaroni and cheese, fried chicken with biscuits, and more. Just talking about those meals takes me back to the days of mindless eating without a care. And when it came to dessert, Mama made the best peanut butter cookies and pound cake on the planet. Everyone loved her pound cake. It tasted like she used at least two pounds of butter. For that reason alone, we should have called it "two pound cake." All that butter made it taste so much better.

One thing is for sure: We ate very well seven days a week. It wasn't just at my mama's house that we ate this way. It was at Grandma's house and our aunts' houses, too. I always ate my fill, but I hardly ever finished all of the food I piled on my plate back then. My brother didn't mind, though, because he got to eat all of my leftovers.

When we weren't eating those delicious meals, my granddaddy used to spoil us with goodies from the gas station where he worked.

He frequently brought home chips, candy, and other special treats. On payday, he gave each of us some money to walk to the store and pick out all of the junk food we wanted. We loved when Granddaddy got paid because Mama only gave us a quarter when we wanted to buy something special. If I asked for fifty cents, it was as if I was trying to rob a bank.

"Mama, it's only fifty cents!" I'd plead.

"Jenny, money doesn't grow on trees!" And then she'd send me off to ask my granddaddy for the money.

Now, *he'd* give us three dollars—each! It felt like I could buy up the whole store with that money. I have always had more of a taste for salty treats than sugary ones, so as a kid I preferred eating pickles and potato chips over candy and cakes. The saltier, the better for me.

As I got older, all of those big meals and all that junk food began to catch up with me. I went from being a skinny chicken to a round and robust young woman. I wasn't fat, but people were no longer seeing my ribs. I was starting to look like the rest of my family.

As I gradually gained weight, I started to develop my own way of dressing. I liked to call it "free style." I chose clothes I liked, not things that were trendy or name brands, which was what my brother and sister always went for. I chose to accentuate my curves, or to just show my personal flair. Some might have thought my outfits were a little weird—but I liked to think of them as unique. I didn't care what size I wore. I just wore what I liked. One of my favorite outfits included a pair of overalls, which I wore to high school at least once a week. I was establishing a personal style . . . and flair, in lots of different ways, something my mama started to notice.

For example, I have always signed my name with great flourish. Even as a child, I made big swoops and grand letters.

"Jenny, you have an artistic signature. I think you can draw!" my mother said with great enthusiasm.

"Whatever," I said.

At the time, I had no interest in drawing. But then, one day, I gave it a try and I've not put my pencil down since. My whole bedroom was covered in my sketches. I have an uncanny ability to draw whatever I see. I always tell people that I got my grandma's voice and my mother's artistic talent.

Then my mother came to me and said, "Jenny, you're such a prankster, I think you might be able to act. I really believe you will be an actress someday."

It's true that as a kid, I was a real practical joker. I loved (and still love) to play tricks on my family and did so whenever I had the chance.

"Whatever," I said.

Do you see a pattern? My usual response of "whatever" turned out to be quite appropriate because *whatever* my mama spoke of *inevitably* came true.

My family always says my voice is a gift—a precious jewel I

inherited from my maternal grandmother. My grandma's name was Julia Kate Hudson. My sister and I used to joke that the Kates in our family got all the talent. (My middle name is Kate, and one of my names in my family is Jenny Kate—which I call myself when I'm just being me, hanging out and doing ordinary things.)

People often spoke about how beautifully my grandmother could sing. She was also the sweetest, kindest, most loving and giving woman. I absolutely loved spending time with her, and especially listening to her sing. She loved to sing hymns and praise God with her voice.

Grandma's house had high ceilings and hardwood floors, which resulted in amazing acoustics. The openness created a sound as if I was singing into a microphone. I would sit on her stairs and just sing my heart out. We have a lot of great singers in our family, so my voice wasn't all that unusual, but some of my older family members told me I had "the gift." They also often said I reminded them of my grandma. I loved to sing and perform. People responded to my voice when I started singing in church or at local talent shows. People would come from all over Chicago just to hear me sing. I became aware that I could move them with my music, and I liked the way that felt. There was a certain sense of power that came with capturing my audience that left me wanting more. They say that most performers live for the applause. Even as a little girl I understood what that meant, and the more I got, the more I wanted.

Even though Grandma had a beautiful voice, she used to tell me that she never wanted to become famous because she'd have to move and perform on demand even if she didn't feel like it—what we would call being "on" today. There are plenty of days performers need to be lifted up and are expected to have the energy to do the lifting. Grandma was perfectly content singing for the Lord. As long as she was reading her Bible or singing in church, she was happy. I remember being mesmerized watching her sing in our church choir. She did more than one hundred solos in that church. Grandma taught me her favorite gospel songs, which I loved to sing. They were powerful and emotional, and everything I thought a song should be to evoke those same reactions from the audience. Grandma's love for gospel is the reason I make sure to have at least one inspirational song on my albums. It is my way of keeping her close, even now.

Around my thirteenth birthday, Grandma had her first stroke and then started having seizures. I never wanted her to be alone so I spent most of my free time keeping her company. I was always quick to volunteer to spend the day at her house so she wouldn't get lonely. There were some good days when Grandma would be up and well, shuffling her feet, singing her hymns; but then there were days when she couldn't get out of bed. Those days were my inspiration to write my first song, called "To Love Somebody," so Grandma would know how much she meant to me. I sat on the side of her bed and sang it to her.

*"It feels good to love somebody, but it hurts to let them go.*
*And it hurts to love somebody when you know*
*you have to let them go."*

Grandma passed away when I was sixteen years old. Since then, I've carried a heart-shaped stone with me wherever I go, as a way to connect to my grandma. I inherited her gift, and I try to keep her memory close.

After Grandma died, instead of wallowing in my sadness, I vowed that I would go on with my life, follow my dream, and make good decisions along the way so I would make her proud. My grandma and mama were the two most important women in my life because they showed me that with the faith of a mustard seed, anything was possible.

In high school, I wasn't what you'd call a typical teenager. I didn't hang out much with girlfriends, other than my friends from choir. I spent most of my free time with my family. I did have a boyfriend, but he went to a different high school and we only saw each other in the neighborhood. My life wasn't full of the typical teenager things like movies and parties and dances and things like that. I was focused, even then, on my music.

I still love spending time with my family and old friends from home. Being with these familiar touchstones helps me to stay grounded. I am still the same person I've always been, which I think surprises people. I remind them that my career doesn't define me. Sure, it's a part of who I am but it doesn't determine how I act.

I do.

I've never forgotten where I came from, so when it comes to family and good friends, bring it on. The more, the merrier. That is why my cousin helps me with my son and one of my brothers works security for me. Even my best friend from middle school, Walter Williams III, works for me as my executive assistant. He's my gatekeeper, and my best friend in the whole world.

Walter and I met in the sixth grade and have been best friends ever since. Even though Walter is slightly older than me, he is still the same height as he was on the day we met—meaning short. I was unusually tall for my age back then. We were quite a pair. We still are.

I will never forget when Walter and I truly connected. There was a new music teacher at our school who wanted to hear each kid sing. I guess she wanted to know what she had to work with. All of the kids in the class pointed toward me, saying, "Jennifer should sing first!" I really had no choice but to do my thing when the teacher asked me to get up to sing.

Up to this point, Walter had never heard my voice. But when I finished, I could tell that he had fallen in love with what he heard. He became my number one fan that day and we've been inseparable ever since. He decided that he would make it his business to make me a star, and I am being honest when I say that I wouldn't be where I am today without his help and support.

Although I had a desire to perform in those early years, I *was* sometimes shy. It was Walter who eventually helped me to come out of my shell. He encouraged me to sing wherever and as often as I could. When we graduated eighth grade, I was asked to sing a solo during the ceremony. I did my own rendition of "Wind Beneath My Wings," and cried through the entire song. Walter and my mama were mad at me for blowing that big moment. In fact, Walter got so upset that he decided he was done with trying to promote my career right then and there. This would mark the first of many times to come that Walter would fire himself out of my life.

After that, Walter and I ended up attending different high schools, but we still saw each other almost every day. We'd go shopping after school, work on music, talk about whom we had crushes on, and just hang out like typical kids our age. We even went to my high school prom together. Walter was my date—he had a car and could drive to the dance. My boyfriend at the time didn't have a car, so he was out and Walter was in. I wore a long cream-colored gown. Every year I have a favorite color, and that year I was in love with anything cream or brown. (This year I'm all about purple, by the way.)

During high school, I took my first job. At the time, my sister was the queen of our local Burger King. Although she wasn't the manager, it was as if she worked that whole place by herself. My sister suggested I come to work with her as a way to make some extra money to support my retail habit—it took money to develop my "free style." I gave it my best shot, but I wasn't cut out for it. The grill was too hot for me! Plus, the manager was not very nice and talked to everyone with disrespect. She may have intimidated the other employees, but not me (or my sister, for that matter). Shortly after I started, I looked the manager square in the eyes and said, "Honey, I am only sixteen years old. I don't need this job! I quit!" My sister gave me a hard time about giving up so quickly, but I knew it was the moment to get serious about what I really wanted to do.

Walter was happy that I quit—and started to work even harder to help me launch my career.

Somewhere around the end of my freshman year of high school, Walter phoned me up and said that he wanted to be my official manager. My first response was a gut-busting laugh, and one of my classic "Whatever"s. But then I said, "All right. You wanna be my manager? Fine!" I figured he would last about a hot minute. Much to my surprise, Walter took his new position very seriously. He started booking shows for me almost right away and escorted me to all of my events. Neither of us could afford to buy the fancy dresses I needed to wear for my gigs. He used his credit card to buy them, and I would wear them once. Walter would then return the outfits for a full refund. Oh, some of those outfits were something

else. Walter did the shopping, and because of my curves we were
limited in where we could shop. One outfit that I may never forgive
Walter for was an orange suit consisting of a jacket and capri pants.
I believe there was some gold trim involved. It was definitely more
of something a grandmother would wear. A very stylish grandma,
but a grandma nonetheless.

Walter even had business cards printed up that read, "Weddings, funerals, and church functions." It also listed my rate of $25
per song in the upper-left corner. Walter's name and number were
on the bottom right as my booking contact.

I'd do my events, get paid, and promptly give Walter his 10
percent. Then we'd return whatever dress we had chosen for the
event. We were making money! For a couple of kids, we thought
we had a pretty good idea of how show business worked. Boy, we
had a lot to learn.

Although I did lots of private parties, my real moneymakers
were competing in talent competitions. There were many talent
shows around Chicago that I could enter. I sometimes wish I could
go back and watch myself onstage. I was pretty confident by this
point. Both Walter and I knew that if I entered, I'd win them all.
We'd look at the prize money and base our decision on which shows
to do on how much money we could make.

I will admit, however, that winning wasn't always easy. You
see, talent shows are a lot like beauty pageants. I felt like I was
under a microscope sometimes, and the atmosphere could be intense

and really competitive. There was so much backstabbing, politics, and dirty tricks going on behind the scenes of those things that I learned to anticipate the *worst* every time we went to a show. I once sang in a competition where another contestant hid my music so I wouldn't be able to perform. This type of sabotage went on all the time. I learned to brush it off and remembered to carry a spare tape.

When I was seventeen, I entered a gospel-singing contest at the mall in Evergreen, Chicago. This was like a local gospel version of *American Idol.* It was one of the biggest competitions in the area. The organizers of the contest had made hair and makeup people available, but Walter had arranged for my own personal glam squad to be with me that day, including a wardrobe stylist, a hair-stylist, and a makeup artist. Walter thought it would be better if I showed up with my own team. It wasn't that we were pulling a diva act. He wanted me to have my own glam squad so I would look the part of a star. My dress that day had been made especially for me by one of Walter's friends. It was a dramatic, black velvet gown, complete with a train and long-fitted sleeves lined with silver fabric.

In an ironic twist of fate, one of the makeup artists provided by the contest organizers is now one of my personal makeup artists.

"I remember you back when you thought you were too good and had your own stylist and hairdresser." She still teases me to this day every chance she gets!

Round one was held at the Evergreen Plaza Shopping Center, and I won. I also won the second round. Like I said, I usually won whatever talent show I entered, and this time I was hoping for the same result.

Round three was held at Salem Baptist Church led by the Reverend James T. Meeks, in Chicago. The church was massive and was by far the largest venue I had ever played. In addition to coming down with a terrible cold, for whatever reason, I switched my song for this round. In the end I don't think I sang the right song to win that contest. I ended up placing third. No matter how big the glam squad, or how dramatic the dress, sometimes things just don't work out.

Walter was always incredibly passionate about ways to move my career in a forward motion. He had the highest expectations for me and would stop at nothing to help me get to the top. One thing I know he wasn't expecting was that I would ever go back to work at Burger King, something I could do only because it was, as they say, "under new management."

This time, I worked the drive-through window. You didn't hear, "Welcome to Burger King. May I take your order" when you drove up to my window. Oh, no. You heard my big ol' mouth singing whatever came to mind. That window had a microphone and I couldn't resist. I have never met a microphone I didn't like—even if it was at a Burger King. I especially loved singing songs from commercials like "... Always, Coca-Cola ..." and even jingles from competitors like McDonald's. That drive-through was my stage and I made sure to entertain our customers as they came by to pick up their Whoppers and fries.

It turned out the new manager of that Burger King was a club promoter on the weekends at a local nightclub called Mr. G's Supperclub & Entertainment Center. Mr. G's was a big deal in Chicago back then. My Burger King manager asked me if I wanted to come down to the club and sing a set or two. He said he could only pay me a hundred and fifty dollars.

*Say what?*

That was a lot more money than I was making working the drive-through or singing at weddings.

I was all over his offer like white on rice.

At the time, I loved listening to Whitney Houston and Destiny's Child, so I figured I could sing a few of their songs and just do my thing. Much to my surprise, the club turned into a regular gig. And just like that, I was done working at Burger King, much to Walter's satisfaction. I made up my mind then and there to make a living by carving out my career using my talents and doing the one thing I love. Working at Burger King was the first and last nine-to-five job I've ever had. I was nineteen years old and have never looked back.

I took general courses while attending college, and naturally, music was one of them. My teacher there was a gentleman named Rufus Hill. On the first day of class, he made each of the students get up and sing for him. I felt like it was grade school all over again! When it was my turn, I sang "His Eye Is on the Sparrow," which was a traditional gospel song I knew I could handle. By the time I finished singing, Mr. Hill was practically on the phone to his friend, a well-known theater coach. He called to have her come hear me sing.

The following week, she came to our classroom so I could sing for her. At the time, I had no idea why, but if someone asked me to perform, I was always happy to oblige. Turned out that she was looking for people to audition for the musical *Big River.* It was being staged at Marriott Theatre in Lincolnshire, about an hour and a half outside of Chicago. I was going to try out.

Mr. Hill and his friend spent the next several weeks helping me prepare for my audition. They worked with me and helped me learn the music and lines. I practiced "How Blest We Are," the most important song from *Big River,* until I knew it cold. I got the part and finally had my first real *professional* singing job.

From that point forward, Walter and I knew we'd ultimately take this journey together. I have always called Walter my life partner because we have been through everything together from the start. He knows me better than I know myself, and he's always believed in me. I personally think every girl ought to have herself at least one gay man in her life because he will always tell you if your shoes are so last season, your outfit is not working for you, your hair is a total wreck, or to get rid of that man you are dating if he isn't treating you right! I always tell people that if they don't like Walter, there isn't something wrong with him—there's something wrong with them!

# CHAPTER TWO

# INVISIBLE

B y the time I was in my teens I was aware that I had become a plus-size girl. C'mon, I wasn't blind. I may never have called myself "fat" but I still knew that I couldn't shop where other girls shopped. I just felt confident that I could work with the body God gave me. I wasn't insecure—I had all the great curves that a lot of women have to pay for!

When I was fourteen years old, I was in a group called Final Notice. The other two girls were a little older than me, and comparatively speaking, they were petite. I was younger and, well, not as delicate. I wasn't overweight, and because of my five-foot-nine frame, I was able to carry a few extra pounds—and carry them well. Even though I didn't fit the look they were going for, they kept me around because I had the most talent. Image was always the bigger issue with the girls in that group. The other girls didn't want what I wanted—which was to sing. They wanted to wear skimpy little outfits so they would look hot. I wanted to choose costumes we could all wear to *entertain*.

The girls from Final Notice and I would go to pick our outfits together, and this was often a frustrating experience. We'd go shopping and I'd try on matching jeans that were supposed to be in my size. While they always fit the other girls perfectly, mine were never quite right. Since I am so tall, I'd usually end up with jeans that were tight in the waist and far too short. If I went up a size, they were baggy all over and made me look even bigger than I was.

Many studies claim that approximately 60 percent of the population is considered overweight. If half of the population is women, then roughly ninety-three million are female shoppers in the double-digit size range. That is a lot of women. Those women are the average, not the exception. I've been one of those women, and I've had many times in my life when I felt like I was not going to find the right things to wear. That's why I got the idea of opening up a clothing store of my own and calling it Average Sizes, because the average woman in America wears a size 14. If the average American woman is a size 14, wouldn't it stand to reason that a size 14 would be the most common size sold? It's not. It seems like sizes 12 and 14 are in fashion hell because manufacturers can't figure out how to make clothes that really appeal to women who are that size. I always hated that most stores carried clothes in small, medium, and large or sizes 0 to 14. If you didn't fit into those sizes, there was a separation that suddenly made you "plus" size and forced you into shopping at places like Fashion Bug and Lane Bryant. I had nothing against these stores. In fact, I was grateful for their existence. I just didn't want to feel different for having to shop there. There was a store near us called 5-7-9, and my sister, Julia, and I used to joke that if you combined those sizes, *that* was a size that would fit us!

There are more options now than there used to be, but there is still some stigma attached to shopping in the plus department or at plus-size stores. And don't get me started on some of the things that designers think plus-size women want to wear. It seems as if they think that the bigger you are, the more sparkles or prints you want on your body. I'm sorry, but why would that be true? Why can't plus-size women just have a nice pair of jeans that fit well, and a great black top that hugs in all the right ways? (This is my note to designers out there—do right by the average woman!)

*Why is it so hard for an average-size woman to find clothes that fit? According to* Women's Wear Daily, *women who used to be a size 8 or 10 and have gained weight often don't want to shop for a size 14 or 16. They end up making do with the clothes they have. Interestingly, women sizes 20 and up, many of whom have likely been plus size their entire lives, seem to be more likely to have accepted themselves physically, and shop as frequently as single-digit-size women.*

Julia once came to a Final Notice show and overheard people talking in the audience, saying, "She can sing but her clothes are too small!" Now, Julia has always been a big girl herself, so she didn't understand why these girls in the audience were commenting on the size of *my* outfits. I was only wearing what the group put me in. The bigger dilemma for me was that I had to conform to their image or I'd be out of the group. We were definitely at a crossroads. Even though I couldn't fit into the clothes they wore most of the time, I was still expected to do all the work in pants that were too tight, too short, and, truthfully, really uncomfortable. The other girls had the look but couldn't sing. This didn't make a lot of sense to me. I moved on.

The next group I was in was called Fate's Cousins, a group I was in with two of my cousins. We picked the name as our way of paying homage to our favorite group at the time, Destiny's Child. Ironically, I was the *smallest* girl in that group. We didn't last very long, but after my experiences with Final Notice, I made sure Fate's Cousins were about one thing and one thing only. *Singing.*

There were plenty of times I auditioned for other groups and didn't get the job because I didn't fit the image. I didn't see this at the time. Then I was just confused, and hurt. I honestly thought that my talent was the thing that should, or should not, secure jobs for me. I didn't fully grasp how important image was in show business. One such experience really sticks out in my memory—when I auditioned to be a backup singer for Barry Manilow. I was nineteen years old and probably at my peak weight of around 236 pounds.

I had never been on an audition where I would have to sing *and* dance. I'll dance if I have to and sometimes when I perform, but I don't necessarily think of myself as a dancer. Still, I'm a professional, and I'll do what is required when it is called for.

The audition went amazingly.

I performed a gospel song called "Silver and Gold." All of the casting people there, including Barry Manilow himself, absolutely loved what they heard. They were crazy excited when I finished. Where I come from, people will throw things at you when they think you did a great job. And when I finished singing that day, everyone in the room was throwing things my way. They picked up whatever they had nearby and tossed it at me so I would know they thought it was great. People in the hallway still waiting to audition were saying they didn't want to follow me. "What's the point?" I heard one girl say.

Oh yeah. I killed it.

I waited in the hallway for someone to come tell me a start date.

"I'm so sorry, Jennifer. We don't have anything for you."

You read that right.

That's exactly what they said.

"Are you kidding me?" I asked.

You could have knocked me over with a feather. Turned out, I didn't have the look so I didn't get the part. I was extremely disappointed. I was dismayed. I thought I had nailed it and the job was mine. It took me years to realize that I didn't get the job because of my size. At the time, I was just upset that I wasn't going to get a chance to share my talents with a larger audience.

The thing I got from these experiences was that not everyone has the same values and focus. My focus has always been on talent over looks. This theme of people putting an emphasis on looks first has been a constant reminder throughout my life that most people don't see things in the same way that I do. Looking back, I realize that it has always been my appearance that I have been judged on first. It made a difference whether I was fat or skinny. This is something I never totally accepted but was learning that I had to deal with.

Coming off of the Barry Manilow disappointment, I was given a challenge. At the time, I was signed to a record deal with a Chicago-based independent label called Righteous Records, headed by a man named David Johnson. He created a contest for me to be inspired to lose the weight, pitting me against another girl on the label who was much smaller than I was. David said we both needed to lose weight and whoever lost the most would win money. I am the type of person who doesn't like being told what she can and cannot do. And if you challenge me, I will accept. And don't expect to win, because I will crush you.

Let me say that I've always been a real girl. If I can't do something naturally, I won't do it at all. Period. So I knew that if I wanted to win this contest, I'd be doing it the old-fashioned way—by working for it.

So I started exercising every day. I'd get up in the morning and do my DVD workouts, first with Billy Blanks's Tae Bo and then aerobics with Denise Austin. Next, I'd go jogging around my neighborhood. I heard that people used to look out their window and ask, "Who's that girl running around out there?" It didn't take long for everyone to figure out it was just me. Next I'd run up and down some local stairs for fifteen minutes and then jog back home. When I wasn't working out around my house, I'd head to the gym.

I started watching what I ate for the first time in my life. I stopped eating fried foods, red meat, pizza, carbonated sodas, and ice cream (all foods I would avoid as a rule until I started Weight Watchers). I went on a total meat-tox, cheese-tox, and sugar-tox. I ate grilled chicken, brown rice, and broccoli—straight-up diet foods. All the time. And nothing else. I did this same exercise routine for the first half of my day—every day—until I lost sixty pounds and got down to a size 10.

To me, being a size 10 was perfect. I thought, surely I could become a star looking like this. Who would have ever believed that size 10 is still considered plus size in Hollywood? Really, I just didn't get it.

Shortly after this first weight loss, Walter came to me and said, "The world needs to hear you, Jen, and I'm going to make sure they do!" God bless Walter because he would go around finding anything I could sing for or be a part of. Walter found out that Disney was holding auditions for cruise-ship singers at a theater school on the northwest side of Chicago. I hadn't sung for anyone in a while. I had been so focused on losing weight and getting myself in shape. To be honest, I wasn't very excited about the audition but I reluctantly agreed to go. Really, I didn't love the idea of taking a job on a cruise ship and traveling so far from home.

But the audition was two days after my birthday, and I had just gotten a new dress I looked fab in. Since Walter was so insistent, I agreed.

Disney hired me on the spot. Interestingly, the casting director told me they would have hired me regardless of how much I weighed. Disney didn't seem to have the same hang-ups about weight and appearances as other entertainment companies I'd auditioned for in the past. They believed in my talent above everything else. I guess I finally fit the bill for that.

It was around this time that *American Idol* was holding its auditions for its second season. Walter and my mama kept telling me I should try out this time. In the summer of 2002, *American Idol* made its television debut. It wasn't yet the phenomenon it is today, so I didn't pay much attention to it that first year. But my mama watched the show all the time. One day she came to me and said, "Jenny, I think you ought to go and audition for this show."

"Whatever," I said . . . again.

I'd already had my fill of talent shows, and truth be told, I wasn't the least bit interested in this one. But by the time Kelly Clarkson was named the first American Idol, I was stunned that something like that could actually happen on television. I was suddenly embarrassed that I had been so cavalier about this show, and started asking myself, "Why didn't I go?" over and over again. I was completely hooked from that point on.

Unsurprisingly, Walter was on me pretty hard about missing that shot at fame.

Even so, I wasn't so sure about auditioning for *American Idol* now. Since I had already been offered the Disney position, I knew that was a sure thing. If I gave that up to audition for *American Idol*, I'd be taking a risk even I wasn't willing to bet on. I figured that I better go with the sure thing. So, I skipped the second year of *American Idol* to work on the cruise ship.

Disney moved me down to Orlando, Florida, for two months of training before I spent the next six months performing on the ship. I was cast as one of the Muses in a production of *Hercules the Musical*, and I also had a solo in *Disney Dreams*, which was a show made up of songs and clips from Disney classics. My song was "The Circle of Life" from *The Lion King*.

The shows were a lot of fun but definitely rigorous and grueling. I had to dance and sing all throughout the productions. Thankfully my weight was in a good place, which made it easier for me to keep up the pace than if I had been heavier.

Doing those shows was so energizing, and the audiences were amazing week after week. There's something wonderful about entertaining people on vacation. Everyone is there to have a good time. Even though I loved performing each night, being on the ship was a little boring, because we'd go to the same places over and over again. I never knew what day it was, because they were all pretty much the same.

I've always been a homebody and a mama's girl, so being away from my family, stuck on a cruise ship, wasn't easy. I'm going to be honest and tell you that two days into my contract I began counting down the days until I could get off the ship and go home. I genuinely missed my family. I lasted the eight months working for Disney, and then I went home. That was enough for me.

In the end, I was extremely grateful for the time I spent on the ship, especially because it gave me the opportunity to save up my pay. I have always been a saver, but living on the ship meant all my meals and living expenses were covered and I could save a lot.

As soon as I got back to Chicago, Walter surprised me with the news that he had arranged for us to go audition for season three of

*American Idol.* He had already bought the plane tickets. There was no way I could back out. Just two days after my return from the cruise ship, he and I headed down to Atlanta, where I would audition among thousands of other hopefuls. And as fate would have it, this is really where it all began.

# CHAPTER THREE

# SPOTLIGHT

Walter and I arrived in Atlanta and headed straight to the Georgia Dome, where the first round of auditions for the 2004 season of *American Idol* were taking place. When we arrived, the show staff gave me a bracelet with a number on it to hold my place. The staff told auditioning hopefuls from the start that if we left or missed our number being called, we would miss our chance to audition.

I didn't have a job to get back to. I could afford to wait for my shot to audition. As the day went on, I could see the line trickle down as one by one people gave up before they even tried.

Basically, the producers wanted us to sleep inside of that dome and wait it out until it was our turn to sing. People had sleeping bags, full camping gear with them. Walter and I only had the tiny blanket and leftover bags of peanuts and pretzels that we took from the airplane. The blanket was hardly big enough to keep either of us warm for the night. We were just not prepared for camping out anywhere, much less on the floor of the Georgia Dome. I also knew I needed some sleep so my voice would be at its best. Thankfully, I had enough money saved to get Walter and myself a hotel room for the night. I also figured my audition number was high enough that I could slip away. I could get a good night's sleep and come back fresh early the next morning for my audition, and that's just what we did. We quietly snuck off-site and slept in a nearby hotel on that first night. Luckily, when we came back the next morning, they hadn't called my number yet.

The second day, while waiting my turn, I sat back and took in everything that was happening around me. Being at the dome was like a dream come true because it was a room full of amazing singers from all over the world. Eleven thousand of them! Even though it's called *American Idol*, I met hopefuls from South America, Canada, and Europe. What was absolutely thrilling was that every person was there for the same reason—to sing. Some of the kids formed choirs and sang off in a corner. Others were running around showing off their skills to one another. While I had an appreciation for all of the talent, I didn't do either. I wanted to wait for my moment. I was going to sing when it counted and that meant for the talent judges. So Walter and I pretty much stayed to ourselves until it was time for me to sing.

The actual audition took place inside the dome, where there were eleven tables spread across the span of the football field. There were people everywhere. It looked like those tables were handing out cheese samples or something like that because of the way organizers quickly moved people in and out. Randy, Paula, and Simon were not a part of this round. They didn't actually come into the process until your final audition—if you made it that far.

When you're called to the field, you are directed to one of the eleven tables where you are asked to sing at the same time as the other ten contestants down the row. It is a little distracting to have eleven people concurrently singing. If you don't have a great ear, you will likely get distracted by the others. And if that happens, you'll get a "Don't call us—we'll call you. Thank you very much, good-bye."

My audition took place very early that morning. I was a little worried that my voice wouldn't be ready, as I hadn't warmed up yet the way I usually did before I sang. But now was my time to show what I could do.

For my audition, I chose an outfit that I thought looked great on me. I was wearing black corduroy fitted pants, a white halter top that was too short so my stomach hung out, a black bra that showed, always a great look, and really big hair. I mean *big* hair. I had done my eyeliner in thick black Cleopatra swoops up to the outer brim of my eyes. I thought I looked fierce and no one could tell me otherwise. Oh, don't get me wrong. Walter tried to talk me out of this look, but I didn't want to hear it. And trust me, there were some *amazing* getups going on in the dome that day. Looking back now, though, I would have definitely changed my hair.

"Hello. My name is Jennifer Hudson."

"And what are you going to sing for us today?" one of the producers asked.

" 'This Empty Place,' by Cissy Houston."

"All right. Go ahead and begin."

I opened up my big mouth and did my thing—belted out that tune. Everyone in the venue heard my audition. When it was over, they all started clapping. I was so flattered, but also shocked that so many people seemed to know the song I had chosen. We're talking about Whitney's mama so I guess I shouldn't have been that surprised. Even so, they asked me if I could sing one more song for them, something more current and familiar. I chose Celine Dion's "The Power of Love," which I thought would show them a big leap in range and a total switch in genre. When I finished that song, I thought I had done really well—but the producers asked me to sing still one more song. This time I chose "Survivor" by Destiny's Child, a song I'd been singing for years and felt very comfortable with.

In the end, I had gone through three eras, genres, and artists. Thank God I did, because it got me through to the next audition phase. When I finished my last song, I was sent to the right, while those who weren't being asked to stay were sent to the left. As I was leaving, I overheard two boys say, "We can't sing after her!" But they did and they made it, too. I met them afterward and shared a good laugh together about their comment.

The second audition meant going back to Atlanta a few weeks later and singing for the executive producers of the show, Nigel Lythgoe, Ken Warwick, and Cecile Frot-Coutaz. That audition took place in a much smaller venue than the dome. The producers told me to do the exact same thing as I had done in my first audition. Meeting the executive producers was significantly more intense than the prior audition. To be honest, at the time I found their presence to be a little intimidating.

But when I sang "The Power of Love," I could see it in their eyes that I would be going on to the next round in the audition process.

The third round of auditions took place in Pasadena, California, which was where I first actually met Randy Jackson, Paula Abdul, and Simon Cowell. I walked into the room wearing a black Versace dress that I had found while shopping in Atlanta during the second audition. It had a hole cut out between my breasts and the belly button, exposing my midriff. Truth be told, I thought it was a good look. I always joked that my *present gut* was simply my *future abs*. I used to walk around patting my stomach telling everyone I had a six-pack. Of course, they couldn't see it, but it was there, just waiting to come out! Funnily, when my audition aired on television, network censors insisted that the cutout in my dress be filled in; this made it look like it was a simple black dress.

Rest assured that I was still rocking my big hair and swoopy eyes. I introduced myself to the judges and told Randy, Paula, and Simon that I had just finished a job singing on a Disney cruise ship.

"We're expecting something more than a cruise-ship performance," Randy said.

I knew just what he meant.

I sang Aretha Franklin's "Share Your Love with Me" for the judges. When I finished, Randy said I was "brilliant. Absolutely brilliant. The best singer I've heard so far."

Paula seconded him, saying, "No doubt about it—you can sing your . . . behind off! You've got an excellent voice."

Simon didn't actually comment at that time. He simply told the judges to vote, and then said, "Jennifer, see you in Hollywood!"

"Yes!" I said as I pumped my fist in the air.

Oh, yeah, I was going to Hollywood.

My mama, my sister, and Walter were waiting for me in the hallway. They were screaming at the top of their lungs when I came out of the room. I was amazed and excited because I had made it. I overheard Ryan Seacrest say, "Now, *that* is how you celebrate."

I was beyond happy. I couldn't believe that I had a chance to be part of this show that had turned Kelly Clarkson and Ruben Studdard into stars overnight. I couldn't believe that Jennifer Hudson, from the South Side of Chicago, was going to get to sing on what was now the most-watched television show in America. I couldn't believe that my voice was going to be heard by millions of people.

I arrived in Los Angeles in early 2004 to start filming season three of *American Idol*. My main goal going into the auditions was to make it far enough to hear Simon tell me I was the best singer he'd seen. I wouldn't stop giving my all in that competition until I could hear him say that. And before all was said and done, I hoped he would. I always set goals for myself so I have something to work toward. This was my goal for *American Idol*.

I ended up in the final twelve by a stroke of luck. I was picked as one of the judges' wild-card contestants. That was the start of what was a very strange experience for me. I went into *American Idol* thinking it was just another talent show, and quickly learned that this was in no way the case. People reacted to my voice, but they also reacted to me and my look and my stage presence. I was starting to realize what an integral part image was to success in Hollywood.

I was grateful when I made it to the final twelve because I was being given a third chance in a single-chance business. I had made it past the executive producers, I had been sent to Hollywood, and now I was in the final round. I had to make the most of it, and put my best foot forward.

The final twelve contestants on *American Idol* have a tremendous opportunity, one unlike any that you can really imagine unless you've done it. The exposure it provides for someone who has a dream to be a performer is unparalleled. But along with the opportunity comes a very packed schedule. We had a lot of long days, so the nine p.m. curfew was not only important, but necessary. By the end of every day, I was very tired.

The final twelve lived together in a large house in the Hollywood Hills. The bedroom for the female contestants was sort of set up like a slumber party. We were all in the same room. I shared a room with Fantasia Barrino, La Toya London, Camile Velasco, and Amy Adams. There was a cook in the house who prepared meals for us, and we ate what was prepared, together. We were together all the time. Sometimes things were tense.

Early on, I remember one of the musical directors from *American Idol* telling me that everything about me was too big. She said my voice was too big, my size was too big, and my personality was too big.

"Isn't that what being a star is?" I asked. "Stars are larger than life!"

I didn't understand her motivation in telling me that. Perhaps she was trying to break me down. Who knows? Clearly, she wasn't a fan. And clearly, this was not another talent show. This was reality.

Once you make the final twelve, the show provides you with a stylist and makeup artist who are there to help you create your signature look. Before that, however, you are completely on your own. Needless to say, some of my choices got some attention. In those early rounds I wore some outfits that probably put the focus on everything but my voice. I was still thinking that my talent should be the thing people concentrated on, but I was now learning that part of "making it" was cultivating a whole package. Obviously my look didn't fit into the right package at this point.

I'll never forget Simon telling me that my conservative white skirt suit reminded him of a "leather nurse look." When I chose to wear a metallic silver jumpsuit, he said I reminded him of "something a Thanksgiving turkey should be wrapped in." I took it in stride, though. I told him not to knock it until he checked it out and then proceeded to model it for him like I was working the runway in a Paris fashion show. Simon also said that I looked "hideous" in my custom-made pink taffeta dress. This was a dress that I had designed myself, and had made for me by a friend. I liked it. But even my sister called to say I looked like I should be on an Easter egg hunt. So, maybe that outfit wasn't my best, but at least the judges said they liked my song that night, and to me, that was the reason I was there.

Look, I'd been through years of cheeky comments about my fashion choices. I endured them from my siblings; I heard them during the Final Notice days. That said, I did sometimes wonder if I would have heard these sorts of things if I was rail thin. I didn't always have the best things to choose from when it came to my outfits—the options weren't there in the way they were for the ladies who wore "normal" sizes. Everyone told me to hide my curves, the very things I loved about my body. Once I had a stylist, it was all about suit jackets and things that covered me up. I found it all so confusing.

Luckily, there was a fan base building for me out there. Their support helped me keep my confidence high. There wasn't much of anything the judges could say that would have made me fold and give up my dream. Believe me; I'd heard much worse than what those judges were dishing out.

When it comes time to pick our songs, each contestant has a certain amount of leeway. We received our category for the week on the Sunday before the show. "This week is country week" or "This week is Motown week." The producers then give you a catalog of music and let you pick your song from that particular selection. Sometimes the producers would direct you toward a specific song, but *mostly* they let you decide on whatever you want to sing.

We'd go into the studio and record our song on Monday so the band could hear the arrangements, which were often different from the original recording, and then they would break it down to fit the allotted time for our performance on the broadcast. A typical *American Idol* performance comes in a little under the four-minute mark. Once the timing had been worked out, we were given until five p.m. the next day, Tuesday, to nail it down. The show aired live Tuesday night. All in all, we really got only two days to learn and perfect our selections before going in front of the cameras and singing for the judges. In that time we also had to pick our "look" for the show and work on our stage presence.

My first night of performing, I sang John Lennon's "Imagine." The world was finally getting to hear me sing. That night was an unbelievable blessing for me because it meant that I had reached that goal. I was overjoyed and overcome with so much emotion that I got very teary standing with Ryan Seacrest afterward. I was living my dream.

Season three was the first season *American Idol* brought in celebrity guest judges to coach us for particular episodes. I had the honor and privilege to work with some of the greatest talents in the music business, such as Sir Elton John, and from the film world, Quentin Tarantino. Elton John was a guest judge during week four. I absolutely loved working with him—we connected from the very start. From the moment we met, he became my mentor, and as it would turn out, after my time on the show he was my biggest advocate.

When Elton came to rehearsals that week, he said he thought I was destined to become the next American Idol. He loved my voice and supported me in a kind and loving way. Of course, I chose "The Circle of Life" as my song that week. I'd sung it many times before while working on the Disney cruise ship, but I had never sung it like I did that week—and that was all due to the guidance I received from its composer, Sir Elton John.

Quentin Tarantino was the celebrity guest judge during week

five on the show producers called "Movie Night." He was apparently a big fan of the show. To be totally honest, I didn't really know who Quentin Tarantino was at that point. I had never seen any of his movies before the producers of *American Idol* said we'd be attending a screening of his latest film, *Kill Bill: Vol. 2*. Believe it or not, I actually fell asleep at the screening. Now, for those of you who have seen *Kill Bill: Vol. 2*, you know it is hardly a movie to put you to sleep. But I was so tired from our nonstop schedule and being on the go, go, go that a dark movie theater became the perfect nap spot.

After the screening, all of the contestants and crew had a reception for Quentin. I still hadn't met him, so I didn't realize that the guy who had asked me what I thought of the movie was actually the director.

"I fell asleep!" I said, completely oblivious to whom I was speaking. Thank goodness Quentin has a great sense of humor because his reaction was simply to laugh. I am hoping he thought I was kidding. Later, when I realized who he was, I figured I blew any chance I had of ever being in a Quentin Tarantino movie. Funny enough, at his request, I auditioned for him several years later. I was told to show up at his house wearing cutoff blue jean shorts and flip-flops. I didn't get the part, but I hope I'll get another chance to work with him one day!

In the end, Quentin loved my performance on the show that week, for which I sang Whitney Houston's "I Have Nothing," later commenting, "Hudson takes on Houston and wins!" That was the highest compliment I could ever imagine because I *love* Whitney Houston. She is one of my greatest musical inspirations and has been for as long as I have been singing. Thanks, Quentin, but Ms. Houston will always be the gold standard. I am just flattered to be compared to her.

My last week on the show, none other than Barry Manilow was the special guest. I was wondering if Barry would remember me. It would be the first time I saw him since my audition to become his backup singer. The audition that I thought I had nailed, only to be disappointed.

Sure enough, when we met again, Barry said, "Don't I know you from somewhere?" When I reminded him, he remembered me and my audition right away, which was really flattering. He said he was glad to finally be working together. That acknowledgment made me better. The fact that he remembered me meant so much. It's experiences like that that keep me from dwelling on the jobs I didn't get or what didn't work out as planned, because I am a true believer that what is supposed to happen will.

My original song choice that week was "All the Time," a song Barry Manilow wrote for Dionne Warwick. I had already made up my mind about my song choice when someone told me that La Toya had decided to do that song, too. So in the end, I ended up singing Barry's "Weekend in New England." We worked hard to create a performance that would wow America and the judges.

Barry wanted to structure the arrangement of the song in the same way he had done for Jennifer Holliday, a singer he said I reminded him of. It was an ironic comparison, given what would happen next, but I had no idea how connected I was to her at that moment. Barry knew that the arrangement he had done for her on this song would work for me, and it was a truly brilliant arrangement. In the end, it was perfect. I sang my heart out; I thought I brought the house down. It turned out that America didn't agree.

On elimination night, as usual, the safe contestants were separated from the bottom three. George Huff was the odd man standing, awaiting his group assignment. Ryan told him to "join the top group" because he was, in fact, also safe. He hesitated as he slowly made his way toward Fantasia, La Toya, and me.

"George, I said step into the *top* group," Ryan said. "You're in the wrong group because tonight, this is our bottom three— Fantasia, Jennifer Hudson, and La Toya London, America!"

The look of total shock came over everyone's faces, including my own, as the crowd booed and screamed in total disapproval. George, obviously confused, slowly walked toward the other group, which was made up of John Stevens, Diana DeGarmo, and Jasmine Trias, leaving us on our own.

Ryan asked each of the judges what they thought had happened.

When it came time for Simon's comments, he started off by saying, "Tongue . . . floor." I knew what he was feeling. But then he pointed out that the others who were safe had earned it. And again, he was right.

In a rare effort not to draw out the final results, Ryan quickly sent La Toya to the couch, where she was safe and would be back to fight for the title the following week, leaving Fantasia and me on the stage anxiously awaiting our fate. We stood there together, holding hands, like we were lifelong best friends. The whole moment was surreal. One of us was definitely going home. We were told that it was the smallest margin ever that separated two contestants in the bottom two, yet enough of a distance to end the journey for one of us, too.

Secretly, I was praying to God, "Let it be me." I was ready. I knew that *American Idol* was a fantastic launching pad. I didn't care if I won or not. As far as I was concerned, my dream had already come true when I was allowed to sing for millions of Americans for those six incredible weeks.

And then it was time for the moment of truth.

Ryan walked over with the results in his hand and said, "The person going home tonight, in a previous show had the highest number of votes but tonight has the lowest. And that person is . . . Jennifer Hudson."

On April 21, 2004, I was the sixth contestant voted off of *American Idol* season three. I wasn't upset. I wasn't disappointed. To be totally honest, I was relieved. I endured so much to be on that show. I was proud of the struggles I went through because I was, and continue to be, a survivor. But it was time for me to take another step.

As I stood watching my farewell video, I realized that there was so much to be grateful for, too. Going in to *American Idol*, your mind is blown, thinking that you are going to be part of this massive television show. But once you are on the inside, you see it is something so much more than just a show. It is like a boot camp for the music business. It gives you tough skin and a realistic opportunity to see what it is like to live that way. It is an amazing chance to live the life of a famous musician, at least for a little while. To the average person on the street, you're a celebrity, because they see you on TV every week. But to the music executives and Hollywood, you are on the bottom, with a lot of work to do to keep rising to the top. I can't imagine being in a place that could have prepared me any better for my career than *American Idol*. I got to meet people like Elton John and I reconnected with Barry Manilow, both of whom became big fans of mine because of the show. And even Simon Cowell inspired me to follow my dreams, despite the fact that he was a pretty tough critic at times.

I knew in my gut that winning *American Idol* wasn't what God had planned for me. I knew I was going to get to sing again, and that I just had to wait for the right opportunity.

When all was said and done, I wasn't expecting to feel so emotional after leaving the studio that night. I actually cried for a few minutes in the limousine on the way back to the *Idol* house after the show, and again the day after my elimination. I wasn't sad to be leaving the show so much as I was disappointed, and more so, I felt like I was disappointing others, like Walter and my family. Plus, there were so many fans who wanted to see me get to the finals. And for their love and support, I will always be eternally grateful because I know in the deepest part of my heart and soul, those fans are the reason I was able to take my leap off the *Idol* stage.

I wiped away those final tears as the limousine swept me off to the airport so I could fly to New York City and do a myriad of press. Since my elimination had caused such an uproar, there were several extra interviews added to my already full schedule. I stayed in New York for about a week answering as many questions as I could about what I thought went wrong. But inside, I was okay with what had happened. It was hard for a lot of people to understand that sentiment, but I was just at peace with it. And when the storm finally died down, I flew back to Chicago and my family.

We started rehearsals for the *American Idol* Tour a couple of days after Fantasia was named the new American Idol. I was really excited to be a part of that experience because I had never even been to a concert and now, here I was—part of one! I had always vowed that the first concert I wanted to go to would be my own. I felt so lucky.

The tour was a real treat. I loved being onstage, singing and giving everything I had to the audiences each night—especially with so many other talented people. Being on that tour was like a dream come true because we could finally be successful, *together*. Listening to George Huff sing gospel, and warmly embracing music with Fantasia and La Toya, was something I will never forget. If I could bring them all back together, I would. Once the tension of the competition had gone away, it was just pure fun.

I'm so lucky to have been able to maintain my relationship with George—he's now one of the backup singers for me on tour! He is such a dear friend. There will always be an inexplicable bond among all of us from season three, which I hope they all feel as much as I do.

After *American Idol*, life was never the same again. I suddenly saw that I was a familiar face to so many strangers. They saw me as famous even though I had barely started my journey. I had, for the first time in my life, real *fans* from outside of Chicago. It was so cool!

At the time, Walter was still acting as my manager. Sharing my voice with others is what I knew I needed to do, so I hit the road on my own, doing club work and other appearances. God bless the gay community, who embraced my act from the very start. For a while there, it seemed like I was always in Atlanta performing at a gay club.

I was only twenty-two years old and I had been on one of the biggest shows on television, on a coast-to-coast tour that I loved, and was now making a pretty good living singing in clubs on the weekends. But I was just getting started.

# CHAPTER FOUR

# WHERE YOU AT

Six months after I finished *American Idol*, I was approached by Ed Whitlow, one of the directors I had worked with on the Disney cruise ship, to record an album. Ed said he knew a producer who had previously worked with *NSYNC in the past and who could work with me on a couple of songs. Ed reminded me of Walter in a lot of ways. He was willing to do whatever it took to get people to hear my voice. So, I left Chicago and moved to Orlando, Florida, to begin work on an album. Ed allowed me to stay at his home while we worked on putting a record deal together for me, and then I went to work in the studio. I had no idea if anyone would ever hear the music we were working on, but I was simply happy to get into the studio.

For several months, the only thing I did was go to the studio and record. I did a few performances whenever they came up. I took a quick trip to Los Angeles to audition for a part in the movie version of *Rent*—which I didn't get. It seemed God had something else in store for me. In the meantime, I kept working.

In Florida, I was a bit off the radar. I also didn't really focus on my weight at all. I ate what I wanted, relaxed when I could. It was like I needed to hit pause after the hectic but great year I had. I just focused on my music and making my first album.

It was around early spring when I began hearing about a buzz in Hollywood that Jennifer Hudson was being considered to play the role of Effie White in the upcoming film adaptation of the highly popular and successful musical *Dreamgirls*. I kept seeing articles and reading blogs that mentioned me for the part, but I hadn't heard from anyone connected to the film. I had no idea why or how the rumor got started. I had never even seen the stage version. I was completely clueless about the story, the music, or its history. I didn't know anything about the character of Effie White. I only knew of Jennifer Holliday, the originator of the role, because Barry Manilow had spoken of her on *American Idol*. I had never even heard her sing, and I certainly hadn't heard Effie's signature song from the show.

As the rumors began to swirl, I needed to find out who Effie White was and why people were saying I was perfect to play her.

Set in the turbulent early 1960s to mid-1970s, the story of *Dreamgirls* follows the rise of three women—Effie, Deena, and

Lorrell, best friends from Chicago (in the movie they're from Detroit), who form a singing group called the Dreamettes. The group goes to New York City to perform in a talent show at the Apollo Theater in Harlem. They don't win the competition, but backstage they meet an ambitious young manager by the name of Curtis Taylor Jr. Curtis gets the group a spot as the backup singers for James "Thunder" Early, though he makes moves for them to eventually break out on their own. Curtis reshapes the group to "cross over" from the R&B genre to the more lucrative and emerging pop music scene. Effie White, who had been the lead singer of the group due to her amazing voice, is sidelined because as a full-figured woman, she doesn't fit the group's image as Curtis sees it. Effie's journey is at the emotional center of the film and the show, as she resents the change in the group and is eventually replaced, only then to have her life spiral downward as her career stalls. But Effie hangs on and eventually finds success and, more important, peace.

Okay, so this was a role I could completely sink my teeth into. I knew exactly how it felt to be judged for your look. I knew what it was like to not get jobs because you didn't fit an "image." I knew what it was like to deal with people who thought there were things more important than talent. This was practically *my* life. This was a role I had to play.

It turned out that the producers of the film were in fact trying to reach me, but since I didn't really have a manager at this point

(Walter had taken a job abroad during this time), no one associated with the film knew how to find me.

At the time, my cousin Marita Hudson was a publicist for *Ebony* magazine. We called ourselves J-Hud and M-Hud. She is well-known in the entertainment industry and everyone knows we are related. Luckily, one of the casting agents made the connection, too, and figured Marita could contact me. They finally put a call in to Marita and asked if she would relay the message that the producers of *Dreamgirls* would like to meet me.

Her phone call to me went something like this:

"Hello?"

"Girl, it's Marita. Some casting people phoned and said they want to fly you to New York to audition for *Dreamgirls*!"

That was all I needed to hear.

"I waited, Jesus—you said it was going to happen and now it is here!" I screamed.

All I had to do now was pick a song to audition with and study the script that the studio sent to me ahead of time. After giving it a lot of thought, I decided to sing "Easy to Be Hard" from *Hair* because it was similar to the music from *Dreamgirls* and it was also from a musical that made it on Broadway. Plus, I thought the song really showcased my vocal ability.

Marita met me in New York so she could accompany me to the audition. A lot about that first audition is a blur, but I went into it thinking that I had to fully encompass the character of Effie. I felt so connected to her—another big girl with a big voice. I wondered if all the women auditioning were full figured. I wondered if the producers were looking for someone with a different look from mine, even though I knew I could fill that role perfectly. I wore a simple black dress and readied my voice.

I'm almost certain that the film's director, Bill Condon, an Oscar winner for his screenplay for *Gods and Monsters* and a nominee for the screenplay adaptation of *Chicago*, and casting director Jay Binder were both there the day I auditioned. Besides that, there isn't much I can recall, except feeling like I had done a really good job.

"If we don't call you by July, you probably didn't get the part," someone said to me before I left.

It was only April. I had to wait three months to see what happened next? That was going to be hard—much harder than results night on *American Idol*. Luckily I could go back to Florida and continue working on my album. And wait for news.

It turned out that 782 other women had auditioned for the role of Effie. The producers were intent on casting a relative unknown actress and searched the country, from Hollywood to Harlem, to find their Effie. All kinds of women, in all shapes and sizes, tried out for that part. Would you believe that the script called for Effie to be much taller and heavier than I was at the time? I guess I didn't have to worry too much about not getting the role because I was too heavy. The irony of that became much clearer to me later.

May came and went, then June and then July—and I received no call. My heart sank with the thought that someone else had gotten the role. I couldn't get Effie out of my head, and I hated thinking that another actress would play her. Had the audition not gone as well as I had thought?

But the producers hadn't cast someone else. On the last day of July I received a call in Florida, telling me that I needed to go to Los Angeles for a second audition. This time they said they wanted me to sing *the* song.

Oh yeah.

*That* song.

The casting department sent me the sheet music so I could prepare for my next audition. I only received part of the song, not the whole thing. I prepared that portion as best as I could. When I got to the audition, much to my surprise, the woman who went just before I did sang the *entire* song. I was panicking because I didn't know the *whole* song. There was no way I could go into that room pretending I knew the entire song without failing. I certainly didn't want to go in making excuses, as that is not my style. So I slowly walked through the doors and into the room, and proceeded to sing the part I knew. Needless to say, this wasn't my finest hour. I was sure they would cross my name off their potential Effie list. I was devastated.

But they didn't.

Bill Condon got word about what had happened with my sheet

music. About a month after that audition, someone called to sign me to a two-week-hold contract. This meant that I could be given the role sometime in the next two weeks, but that they weren't obligated in any way to hire me. Also, for those two weeks, I couldn't agree to do anything else. Of course, I quickly signed. Once again, I had been given another chance in a one-chance business. I couldn't believe how blessed I was.

Those two weeks were pure torture. I was on pins and needles the whole time. I was so close . . . and yet I still felt so far. Nearly six months had lapsed since I first received the call to audition. They literally waited until the very last second to call. But they called.

I was once again asked to come out to Los Angeles, this time for a screen test. In fact, they asked me to drop everything and hop on a flight that same day.

"And, Jennifer, this time, bring enough stuff with you in case you're asked to stay."

"How much stuff is that?" I asked.

"Everything you own."

I ran out of the recording studio, drove home as fast as I could so I could quickly pack and make my flight. Somewhere in the middle of that hurricane moment, I got a fax of the full sheet music for "And I Am Telling You I'm Not Going" so I could learn the entire song. By the time those wheels touched down in La-La Land, I needed to know that baby inside and out.

I spent the entire six-hour flight singing to myself. I didn't care who heard me or what they thought. I'd occasionally apologize for disrupting the other passengers, but I knew what I had to do. I had to focus on my goal. I had to keep the faith and not let anything get in the way of the job in front to me. I am sure there were a few people on board who recognized me from *American Idol*, but there were many more praying to God I'd shut my big mouth!

By the time we landed, it was very late at night. I went straight to bed so I would be well rested for my big day ahead. I woke up extra early the next morning, so excited to get to the audition that I was nearly jumping out of my skin.

I called my mama before heading to the studio. Being the good mama that she was, she said, "If some things don't work out and you don't get it, then that is okay because something else, something bigger will come."

I heard her and understood why she was saying that to me, so on the ride over, I kept telling myself, "If it's meant for me, it will be." Those words are my mantra in life, and they have never let me down.

It soon became painfully obvious to me that my purpose for being in L.A. was not just another audition. This was a screen test—the last stop, the final step to getting the coveted part. I knew all the other big roles had been cast at this point. If I was cast as Effie, I'd be working alongside a roster of incredible talents—Jamie Foxx, Danny Glover, Beyoncé Knowles, and Eddie Murphy—just to name a few.

I was completely green at this point in my career. I had never had a screen test before. It was like being under a microscope, and I'd be lying if I told you that I didn't feel self-conscious. The screen test took almost six hours. First, they dressed me as Effie, did my hair and makeup so I would look like Effie, and then checked every bit of my appearance. And I mean every bit. They shot my profile from every possible angle, looking at my body from head to toe. I felt scrutinized in a way that I never had before. This was like *American Idol* times a million. I felt like every inch of my body was on display.

When they finished shooting my screen test, the producers brought me into a room and asked me to do the pivotal scene where Effie sings her big song. I did this over and over and over again.

After several hours, I heard someone in the room whisper, "Her voice is the only one that has sustained the entire time."

I did the best I could and gave it my very best effort. And before I left the studio, I was told I would be going home.

I got on a plane and went back to Orlando.

I wasn't sure what to make of this. I didn't have the part yet. But no one else did, either. So, when I walked through my front door, I placed my suitcase in the middle of the floor on the landing as a show of faith. I didn't unpack a thing. I would just wait for them to call me back. I really hoped they would.

By the following morning, I was already back in the studio recording my album. It was a weekend, so our regular crew wasn't there. I was in the booth recording when I heard that I had a phone call. I instinctively knew it was about the movie. I stepped outside to take the call. I stood still, waiting to hear my fate.

"Jennifer Hudson . . ." It was Bill Condon calling. He spoke slowly and methodically, as if he was about to deliver a verdict in a courtroom.

I was barely breathing, waiting with fantastic anticipation as my heart lay on the ground.

"Jennifer Hudson, I called to tell you that you are Effie White!"

"WOOOOOOOO!" I let out a scream of relief that turned to tears of sheer joy.

I did it! I made it!

I fell to my knees and cried. I was so relieved and overwhelmed and thrilled and thankful.

Bill asked me to get on a flight that same day. Of course, I said I would.

I've been gone ever since.

# CHAPTER FIVE

# I'M YOUR *DREAMGIRL* . . .

When I got the role as Effie in *Dreamgirls,* I had never done any professional acting. On the flight to Los Angeles, I kept reminding myself of this blessing God had given me. My grandma used to praise the Lord and say, "How great thou art!" She was talking about the wonders of God's love and His glory. Looking out the window of my plane I realized that, perhaps for the first time in my life, I truly understood what she meant. She was talking about the wonders of this world, wonders that I was now going to see. I cried tears of joy for most of that flight.

One of the first things I found out when I got to Los Angeles to start shooting was that in order to take this role, I was going to have to *gain* weight. You read that right. Gain weight! The script called for Effie to be heavier than I was at the time, and I needed to put on some pounds. Needless to say, I was pretty surprised. So many times I had felt judged for being too big, had lost jobs because I didn't fit the image required. And now, for the first time ever, I was told I was *too small*! Who gets a job in Hollywood and has to *gain* weight?

Me!

I was told to put on an extra twenty pounds before shooting started so I could really look like Effie as the director wanted her to appear. By gaining the weight, I wouldn't have to wear padded costumes or anything. I could be more "natural." Okay, I thought. I know how to do this—I can put on pounds if that is what was required. I launched into a diet of cookies, cakes, and pies all day, every day.

In addition to my new eating regimen, I started rehearsals right away, too. Every day I would walk around the studios like a high school student going to class, with my backpack slung over my shoulder, full of all the different clothes I would need. I went from dance class to vocal class to acting class. I was constantly on the go. In fact, there was so much physical activity during rehearsals that despite my carb-heavy, sugar-laden diet, I started losing weight. The producers quickly noticed my weight loss and told me I needed to focus on gaining. I kicked up my intake a notch and continued to load up on calories, so I could keep on the pounds despite my very active schedule. It wasn't easy, but I knew I couldn't disappoint the producers.

The film officially started shooting on January 9, 2006. Being on the set of *Dreamgirls* was nothing short of—well, a dream come true. First, I actually got to be in this film, and second, I was set to work with some of the biggest stars on the planet. Eddie Murphy, Danny Glover—these were actors I grew up watching. I had been a big Destiny's Child fan, so it was a thrill to work with Beyoncé. And none other than Jamie Foxx, who had just won an Oscar for his amazing performance as Ray Charles, was going to be my love interest. The first time I met Jamie was on the set. We had never said so much as a hello to each other before that first scene together. After doing *American Idol*, I had made a personal promise that I would never let anyone ever intimidate me again. But Lord help me, the first time I met Jamie, I was scared. He walked onto the set and the director said, "Action. . . . Okay, kiss!"

*Huh?* I thought. I was shocked. I was hoping Jamie and I would at least be introduced before we launched into a kissing scene! Oh well, I had a job to do. And luckily, Jamie had done this all a few times before, so he did his best to make me feel comfortable. Here I was, an actress playing her first scene, and I had to kiss Jamie Foxx square on the mouth.

As filming continued, I remember thinking my grandma would have loved seeing all that was happening to me.

"Look, Grandma. Look at what I am doing." I had conversations with her in my head, especially while listening to the music from *Dreamgirls*.

Whenever I wasn't singing or dancing, I wore my headphones, learning the songs for the movie. I would listen closely to those songs, and ask myself the question that I always ask when I'm learning new music: "What is the message I am trying to get across? What does this song mean?" I need to feel the meaning of the song to be able to perform it with emotion. Music always means something. Music is powerful. It can be both spiritual and emotional. My grandmother taught me that all great singers sing with purpose. For this movie, every song had a purpose in that it propelled the story forward. The songs were almost as important as the dialogue—especially for Effie, who was the girl known for her amazing voice. Effie shared her heartache, her joys through singing. If I was going to play Effie with all my heart, I had to do the same. I certainly used that approach when it came time to do my big scene.

Whenever "And I Am Telling You I'm Not Going" came on my headphones, it felt as if the ghost of my grandma was singing in my ears. I could hear her shouting praise and singing gospel like I was seven years old again watching her in church. Once I started singing the song, it was as if she could see me. Feeling her presence helped me find my emotion to power through that very challenging scene.

I have a cousin who once told me not to sing *at* a song, but to just sing the song—and there is a difference. I sink my teeth into a song and attack it like Jaws. If I can't feel the song when I'm singing it, how can I expect the listener to? Every song tells a story. My job is to be the storyteller. I knew that was exactly what I needed to do going into my big scene—I had to own it and make it mine.

My mama used to tell me that she thought I usually worked best under pressure. I never noticed that about myself, but she sure did. When I was a little girl, I used to run around our family church begging for my first solo. When the pastor finally gave me that chance, I was terrified. It was like I was on the edge of a nervous breakdown. But, I also remember feeling a certain exhilarating electricity about it, too. Those feelings are what gave me the presence of mind I needed when it came time to sing in front of a crowd. I became addicted to the anxiety of performing every bit as much as the thrill of it. Now, when I don't have that sense of panic before performing, I worry about being too calm.

I was anything but calm when it came time to film "And I Am Telling You I'm Not Going." That song is part of one of the most important scenes in the movie. I am not sure I really understood just how big it actually was until after we finished filming. It didn't register until after I completed the scene that I, an unknown actress, had been given the role of a lifetime. The lyrics "And you're gonna love me . . ." were especially poignant because for me, they marked my return to the world stage after my time on *American Idol*. I felt like I was being given a huge chance to send a message out to the world about what I could really do. Truly, I was overwhelmed.

Not knowing the impact of that scene at the time is probably what helped get me through it. What I did know all too well was how Effie felt in that moment after being told she had to leave the group because she didn't fit the image. Lord knows I had been there too many times myself. This was my story every bit as much as it was Effie's. For things to be real, they have to come from a real place. I had lived these moments myself, more than once, and now I could bring all of my past rejection, pain, anger, confusion, and frustration to life through Effie White.

The day we shot my big scene, the set was full of lots of people I didn't recognize—from drivers to crew. Spike Lee and Jamie Foxx came to watch me. When I did my first take, I felt a little self-conscious with so many eyes watching. It was a little like singing in the shower, and turning around to find a bathroom full of people. Luckily, that feeling didn't last very long. By the time I got through that first take, it didn't matter who was there—as far as I was concerned, it was just Grandma and me. I was Effie, and I was feeling her pain.

People gathered all day long to watch. One by one, I could see tears in most everyone's eyes as I sang straight from my gut take after take after take. By the end of the first day, my head was pounding, I was emotionally exhausted and I wanted to rest. Surely, I thought, they had captured the footage they needed. But Bill Condon, being the brilliant filmmaker that he is, knew I could give more. So we continued with the same hard push the entire next day until we got exactly what was needed.

The scene took two whole days to shoot. It felt like the people I saw going into the studio were coming back for their next shift, just as I was leaving. It was an emotional roller-coaster ride for those two days, to say the least. We did the scene over and over again. At times, I felt I had no more to give. I'd start to cry, asking the director what more he wanted from me. I felt tapped out. I was tired. At one point, Bill actually had to tell me to pull back the emotion because I was crying too much for the scene to feel real. At the end of my final take, Bill announced, "Ladies and gentlemen, the star of tomorrow, Ms. Jennifer Hudson." I had to wipe the tears from my tired and weary eyes as the entire studio burst into applause for me. I was overcome.

Without knowing it then, what happened that day created a path for me that I could never have imagined. This day marked a transition in my life, from struggling singer and performer to film actress. I don't think anyone in that studio really understood what had happened that day, and certainly not me. Bill Condon may have. Looking back on that moment now with clear eyes, I know that my life changed forever that day.

I had never acted before this movie, so no one knew what to expect. I was an unknown actress who had been given the role of a lifetime. I felt a real shift in the way I was perceived on the set, a shift that was a nod of approval from my colleagues that I felt happy to receive.

Jamie Foxx was the first person to actually say something about what had happened to me.

"Jennifer, you could get an Oscar nod for this," he said.

Those were big words coming from Jamie Foxx, an Oscar winner himself. The thought of winning awards for my first acting role certainly had not crossed my mind at all.

"Whatever!" I said to Jamie, just like I was talking to my mama. Me and my "whatever"s.

I remember getting a call one day asking me to come to the offices of the studio making the film, DreamWorks, the production company founded by Jeffrey Katzenberg, Steven Spielberg, and David Geffen. David Geffen owned the film rights to *Dreamgirls*, and was one of the producers on the film.

What do they want to talk to *me* about? I wondered. I worried that the producers were concerned about my performance. I felt a little like I was being called to the principal's office. It turned out to be just the opposite. I was told that the buzz on the film was very good, and that Beyoncé, Jamie Foxx, Anika Noni Rose, and I would be attending the 2006 Cannes International Film Festival in May to promote the movie. Cannes? France? I had heard of the festival before, but I never dreamed I'd actually be going there. I was thrilled but nervous, too. I had no idea what kind of appearance I was expected to make. There were going to be numerous grand red-carpet moments, where I would be photographed with some of the most famous people in the world. This was the big time, not like the events that I had attended with *American Idol*, but a huge industry gathering.

The press attending the film festival was going to be given an opportunity to see twenty minutes of never-before-seen footage from *Dreamgirls*. In addition, the press was invited to go "behind the scenes" and meet some of the talent involved in the making of the movie. It was all fantastic.

After Cannes, I started to realize that things were really going to change in my life once this film was released. When I was in the studio recording the sound track for *Dreamgirls*, Beyoncé offered me some advice I've never forgotten. She said, "The way you are starting your acting career is an amazing opportunity for you. Don't hop at just anything. You will have a lot coming at you. Take your time and make the right decisions." These were important words of wisdom coming from a woman I very much admired and respected. At the time, I didn't realize just how amazing the opportunity to play Effie was for me. But I do now, and I have lived by Beyoncé's advice ever since.

The biggest moment for me before *Dreamgirls* was released was one day when I received a phone call from none other than Oprah. You know, Winfrey. I was in a hotel room in New York City when someone from her staff called ahead to let me know she would be calling me later that day. I guess they didn't want me to be taken off guard. Instead, I just didn't believe them.

Whatever, I thought.

I mean, why would Oprah be calling me? I actually thought it was a practical joke someone was playing.

Me and my "whatever"s strike again.

But Oprah did call me the next day. My makeup artist answered the phone.

"Oprah's on the phone," she said.

Now, I was *sure* this was a joke, so I decided to play along.

"Hello?" I said in a disbelieving tone.

"Hi, this is Oprah," the voice on the other end of the phone said.

I didn't believe it was her. "This isn't Oprah," I said, and then I hung up the phone.

I have to believe this happens to her a lot because she called right back and laughingly said, "It is Oprah, like, for real!"

"Girl, I don't know who you are but stop playing with me!" I said. Before I could slam down the phone again, Oprah repeated that it was really her. She was calling to congratulate me on the movie. She had seen an advanced screening and said she was blown away by my performance, calling it "a religious experience."

*Wow!*

That's about all you can really say after hearing something like that from Ms. Oprah Winfrey. That phone call was the beginning of a much-cherished relationship I now have with "Mama O." I always tease her and say that she is the queen and I am a princess. Oprah is one of the few people I've come to know through my career who will take the time to talk to me and tell it to me like it is.

Whether I want to hear it or not, Oprah tells the truth. And if you're smart, you'll listen. I say a lot of "Yes, ma'am"s when we get together. Oprah will say what she has to say *one* time. She's not out to convince me of anything other than that her heart is always in the right place. It is up to me to accept what she says or not. And let me say that when Oprah talks, I listen, because she has a lifetime of insights and experience ahead of me that I would be foolish to ignore. Oprah reminds me so much of my own mother, because that is exactly the way Mama was with me, too.

So, I had played my first role in a feature film, the role of a lifetime. I had been to Cannes. I had been told I could get an Oscar nod for the work I did. I had received a call of congratulations from Ms. Oprah Winfrey. What more could a girl ask for? I was already blessed beyond my wildest dreams. But more was coming, more than I could imagine.

# CHAPTER SIX

# AND I AM TELLING YOU I'M NOT GOING

After Cannes, the buzz on *Dreamgirls* really got going. I was feeling so much love from Hollywood, something I was completely not prepared for. It was all really flattering, but also a little confusing and overwhelming at the same time. The big girl with the big voice was getting congratulated on her success, and not told that she had to lose weight to fit the right image for a celebrity. I thought that sentiment would last, but just in case, I tried to enjoy it for as long as I could.

After the movie wrapped production I went back home to Chicago for the summer and tried to get back to life as I once knew it. I lost the twenty pounds I had gained for the film doing what I had always done—eating brown rice, chicken, and broccoli, and getting up every day at five a.m. to run. I was back on the same cycle that had worked for me before. I spent that entire summer work-ing out on my own in the morning, and then again at a local gym in the afternoon. I was doing what basketball players refer to as "two-a-days." I thought I was doing everything right, eating the right things, exercising the right way. My system was effective, because by the end of the summer, I got right back to where I always landed—a comfortable size 10.

I continued working on my album, spending most of my spare time recording in the studio. Sometime toward the end of the sum-mer, the producers of *Dreamgirls* called to say they wanted me to come back to Los Angeles to do some pickup shots they needed to finish the film. Pickups are small or minor shots that are filmed after a movie is wrapped to augment existing footage. This some-times is needed when the right shot isn't available during the editing process or when the studio wants to tweak a scene because it doesn't play well once they've put the pieces together. I was happy to do whatever they needed me to do, of course. In fact, I was happy to step back into the role of Effie.

And then they dropped a real bomb.

"You have to gain back all of the weight you've lost," the pro-ducers said.

I didn't even have to think about it. "No way," was my response.

I had worked hard to lose those twenty pounds. Too hard to pack them back on again. I was feeling good, back in my size-10 clothes. I thought I looked good, too. Plus, gaining that much weight in such a short amount of time couldn't possibly be healthy. They only needed me to do one or two quick shots. Surely they would be able to work something out without me having to gain back all of the weight I had just dropped! I stood my ground, and though it was a bit of a struggle, the studio finally let it go. They solved the problem by shooting close-ups of me, so the audience could not see the difference in my body.

Back in Cannes, I had been introduced to a Hollywood agent at the special screening for the film set up by the studio. After the movie ended, she came over to talk to me.

"Has Clive Davis ever heard you sing?" she asked.

As far as I knew, the answer was no. Clive Davis is the legendary music producer and musical genius behind the careers of so many talented singers, including Whitney Houston, Alicia Keys, and Kelly Clarkson, just to name a few. The agent assured me that as soon as she got back to the United States, she would go straight to his office and tell him all about me. I figured I'd wait and see if that really happened. I thought that I was in the right place to meet the kind of person who could make such a fantastic connection for me, so I felt cautiously optimistic.

By November 2006, Clive Davis had bought out my existing recording contract with another label and signed me to Arista Records. Clive took me under his wing and has treated me like a daughter from day one. In his own way, Clive let me know that I didn't stand a chance of becoming a superstar performer if I stayed "fat." It was actually Walter who shared this with me. I think he dreaded saying it to me, but as my best friend, he knew he had to. My response was, "When was someone going to tell me?" But as tough as it was to hear, I knew it was tough love coming from Clive Davis. I also knew that Clive Davis understood the music business far better than I did. I also knew that he had an understanding that image sets the standard in the record industry. If Clive doesn't like your image, he isn't signing you. So the fact that he believed in me enough to say what he said made me take it to heart.

I announced my record deal on *The Oprah Winfrey Show,* where I shared my plans to get into the studio to record my *official* "first" album in early 2007. It was during that same show that I received a videotaped apology from none other than Mr. Simon Cowell for being so tough on me on *American Idol.* "Don't forget to thank me in your Oscar acceptance speech!" he joked. To be honest, though, I had never harbored one moment of anger or disrespect for Simon or any of the other judges from that show. They did exactly what they were supposed to do. They offered advice, which was mine to accept or reject. I was eternally grateful for the chance to be on *American Idol,* now more than ever, because I know I got to stand before the world as Effie White because of the chance that show gave me to sing in front of millions of people.

was so excited to start work on my first real record, but before I could do that *Dreamgirls* was going to open, and I would see myself on the big screen for the first time. Just before the world-wide premiere of *Dreamgirls*, the reality of what had happened suddenly hit me. It was early December 2006. I was sitting in a parking lot one night just thinking, *Oh my God.* I just did a major motion picture. I got the part of Effie White and the world is about to see what I can really do. I have a record deal with Arista and Clive Davis. I am beyond fortunate. What else could be in store for me?

*Dreamgirls* had a limited opening in theaters on December 22, 2006, and its national release on January 12, 2007. Studios will sometimes release a film early in a small number of theaters so it can be considered for the upcoming awards season, and Dream-Works had high hopes for *Dreamgirls*.

In the fall, I attended premieres for the film in New York, Los Angeles, and London. These evenings were amazing, like a dream. I wore gorgeous gowns, walked the red carpet, and tried to live in these once-in-a-lifetime moments. Not once during any of the pre-mieres did I hear a single comment about my look. I hoped those days were behind me.

I wanted to watch the film with regular moviegoers, not with just my family or other industry professionals, to see what it was like. The first time I watched the film with strangers was around Christmas. Julia, Jason, and I went to a theater in my old neighborhood in Chicago and snuck in after the film started so no one would know I was there. We stood off to the side and watched the audience's reactions. I was dying inside, waiting for that moment when I sing "And I Am Telling You I'm Not Going." I knew what that scene meant to me because of the way I had connected to the emotions to create that moment, but I had no idea how regular folks would react. It was like being naked and exposed up there with hundreds of eyes watching and judging me. When the time finally came for that scene, I wanted to crawl under a chair and hide. Thank God my brother and sister were there.

On the heels of my last note, everyone in the audience stood from their chairs and clapped. I got a standing ovation—in a movie theater!

I was stunned by their response. Absolutely, positively taken aback.

It was so honest, so real. It was a completely different type of applause than I had ever received. It was tender, moving, and fulfilling in every way. I was emotional but very happy.

I will never forget that experience because it opened my eyes to the journey I was taking in a way I couldn't otherwise understand or see until that moment. If it weren't for the fans' reactions and their support, I am not sure I would be where I am today. And for that, I will be forever appreciative and grateful.

*Dreamgirls* was an instant smash hit with both audiences and the press. I was being called the breakout star of the film for my role as Effie White. The studio called to tell me they were going to put a big push behind me for the Academy Awards category of Best Supporting Actress. I could hardly believe what I was hearing.

Were they really talking about me?

Jennifer Hudson . . . Academy Award–nominated *actress*?

Singer, I could wrap my head around. But this was difficult to comprehend.

By mid-January, I attended my first press event in New York City to kick off awards season. I was back to my regular low point of size 10, and feeling really good. I stood in the middle of a large room filled with members of the press, all there to see the breakout star from *Dreamgirls*. Suddenly, someone turned to me and said, "Wait a minute. Who is this? This is not Effie!" I was stunned. Was I *that* unrecognizable? I had lost only twenty pounds!

As I was leaving the event, my publicist turned to me and said, "The producers really want you to gain back the weight. You no longer look like Effie. The press and media feels connected to Effie. If you want their support, you have to get into character."

I was shocked. First of all, the irony of the situation was almost too much to take. I remembered the comments about my weight during

*American Idol.* I remembered not getting the Barry Manilow job. I remembered the comments from the audience during my Final Notice days about my outfits not fitting. Now here I was in Hollywood, in a town where a size 10 is considered plus size, and I was being told to put *on* weight! I had been lauded for my role as Effie. Why couldn't my performance speak for itself? Why did what the scale said when I stepped on it *always* come into play, either one way or the other? I was at my comfortable size. I couldn't win for losing. Literally.

"They want me to do what?" I asked. My publicist could see that I wasn't at all happy with the request. She explained the process of the awards season—Golden Globes to Oscars. She explained that everyone wanted to see Effie. Not Jennifer.

"It's not going to happen," I said to my publicist.

"You are the leading contender, Jennifer. You have the potential to win every award you're nominated for. You don't want to do anything to affect your chances, do you?"

I told her, "It is what it is." And even though I knew it was a risk, I stuck to my guns. Oh, yes. Jenny Kate had made a decision. I was so tired of losing and gaining weight to please other people. I was going to let my work speak for itself.


I had learned a lot of lessons over the years, but especially since my time on *American Idol.* They are the two notions I cling to always—and you've heard me refer to them before in this book.

They are:

**1. If it is meant for me, it will be.**

**2. The talent should speak for itself.**

I was done being judged for my appearance. It shouldn't matter if I weighed the same, fifty pounds more, or a hundred pounds less. Effie was a *character* I *played*. When I look back at pictures of me as Effie, I see a heavier version of me, but she wasn't me. I thought the difference in my appearance only helped to show off my range and commitment as an actress. I wanted people to understand that Effie isn't Jennifer and Jennifer isn't Effie. I certainly didn't want to get pigeonholed as a plus-size actress. I wanted to demonstrate that I did what I had to do to play Effie, but now I was moving forward with other plans. And my gamble paid off because despite my weight at the time, I was nominated for an Oscar after all.

I transformed my look all throughout awards season. For the Golden Globes, I left my hair down in soft waves and wore a navy blue Vera Wang gown with a deep V-neck that twisted at my waist. I was going for old Hollywood glamour that night, and I felt truly glamorous when I received my award for Best Supporting Actress.

Then came the Grammys, which I attended for the first time in February 2007. I was asked that night to present an award with

Justin Timberlake. I chose a tight red dress that I knew really showed off my curves. This was Jennifer's big night out. That night I was J-Hud! I loved that look and felt like I was showing off who I really was outside of Effie White.

And finally, on February 25, 2007, after a whirlwind of accolades, I won the Academy Award for Best Supporting Actress.

When George Clooney announced, "And the Oscar goes to Jennifer Hudson!" I was frozen in my seat. I was positive that I was the only one who heard my name. But then everyone was looking at me in a strange way, clapping and waiting for me to do something. Bill Condon, who escorted me to the awards ceremony that evening and who was sitting next to me, hit me to get up.

"Huh? I just won?" It was the most surreal experience of my life.

When I got to the stage, I had to pause, take a step back, and soak up that moment.

As I began my acceptance speech, thoughts of my grandma came to my mind. That's when I exclaimed her poignant words I'd heard so many times as a child: "Look at what God can do!"

Grandma would have been shouting God's glory across the stage and into the theater. Everything she said to me growing up was suddenly so very real. I really didn't think I was going to win that night, so I did my very best to thank everyone who had helped me keep the faith even when I didn't.

So here it was, almost three years after being voted off *Ameri-*

*can Idol,* and I was now an Academy Award–winning actress. It was almost too much to take.

In an unfortunate twist, I made many "worst dressed at the Oscars" lists. To be truthful, I wasn't very happy with the dress that I wore that night, a brown high-waisted gown paired with a python bolero jacket with a prominent collar. It was not something I ever would have chosen for myself. But I was still pretty new to the Hollywood game. I wore what I had been committed to wear, by someone else and without my knowledge. Let me tell you—that was the last time that happened! I would never again wear something I didn't love 100 percent.

Winning the Oscar opened up the floodgates for more acting opportunities in Hollywood. Movie offers came pouring in. Some were interesting, while others weren't right for me at all. I remembered back to what Beyoncé had told me and carefully considered each before saying yes or no. When the producers of the movie *Precious* asked me to play the title role, I knew it was an amazing role. But I also knew that I would have to again gain a lot of weight to play her. I had done that with Effie, and as much as I was moved by this film, I wanted to try a role that had nothing at all to do with my weight. I turned down *Precious,* and the role went to Gabourey Sidibe. She gave an unforgettable performance in the film, was nominated for an Oscar herself, and the career of another unknown actress was launched.

One movie I did say yes to was *Sex and the City.* I played Carrie Bradshaw's assistant, Louise. This fantastic ensemble cast had been doing their show together for years, so it was a real honor to be asked to become a part of their tight-knit family. It was also a little like being the new kid at school. The cast members of *Sex and the City* are fashion icons, each known for a distinctive, often trendsetting look. I was a little intimidated about how I was going to fit into all of that. I quickly found my stride, and ended up really enjoying playing Louise alongside SJP, as Sarah Jessica Parker is often called.

Doing *Sex and the City* was a really great experience and very different from doing *Dreamgirls.* This set was very fast-paced. The cast members of *Sex and the City* had a long-established groove after years of doing the television show, and they moved each scene right along. While *Dreamgirls* was shot primarily on a soundstage in Los Angeles, *Sex and the City* took place on the streets of New York City. I spent three months living and working in Manhattan, and loved every minute of it. I even got to record "All Dressed in Love," an original song for the movie sound track.

During the time I was filming *Sex and the City,* I began taking notice of a very handsome actor named David Otunga. I told Walter, "Oh, I would love to meet that guy." But I knew that if it was meant to be, it would happen, so I wasn't going to pursue him.

Luckily, things fell into place, and David and I met. I couldn't have been more surprised when I realized he was the *one*.

I had certainly been bitten by the acting bug, but my heart still belonged to making music. As much as I enjoyed acting, I thought it was time to put my focus back on my first true love—singing—and my new love—David.

# CHAPTER SEVEN

# GIVING MYSELF

September 2008 was a very special time in my life. There were two unforgettable moments that altered the course of my life forever. The first was the impending release of my debut album. But before we get to the actual release, let me take you back to how it all came about.

A week after winning my Oscar, I was in the recording studio working on the album. It was almost as if I had to be reintroduced to myself because the last year or so of my life had been such a whirl-wind: singer to actress and back again. I knew there had been a shift in my persona to the world. To almost everyone, I was now thought of as an actress first. I had always been a singer first and foremost.

Clive Davis had taken a very active role in my album and in my career, and this was a great feeling. I also knew that I was going to have to listen closely to what he had to say. I don't always take it well when someone tries to tell me what to do, especially when it comes to my music. However, when that "someone" happens to be Clive Davis, I listen. He's the pro. I was lucky that I got to have a little more freedom than most first-time recording artists, something I didn't take lightly at all. I spoke up when I felt I needed to, and listened to Clive and others when that felt right.

It took me two years to complete my first album, due in part to the fact that out of the gate we had no idea which direction to go in. Coming from singing on *American Idol* and then to *Dreamgirls*, my audience was vast and varied. The musical landscape I was entering was very much in flux. I had a hard time choosing the right songs that would appeal to my audience, but also remain true to my voice and what I think I do best. I like to do big, sweeping ballads, full of emotion and feeling. When you turned on the radio in 2007 and 2008, you didn't really hear songs like that. It was strange to hear Akon's "Smack That" or Amy Winehouse sing "Rehab" followed up by "And I Am Telling You . . ." on the radio. I knew my audience was out there. It was just going to take some time to make the right music for them.

I recorded somewhere around sixty songs over the course of the next two years to pick the final thirteen that ultimately made the album. I took my time recording because I wanted it to be great, for my fans and for me. I thought the fans deserved to have the very best, and you never get a second chance to make your first album. I worked with several different producers and songwriters, including

Ne-Yo, Missy Elliott, Robin Thicke, T-Pain, Tank, Timbaland, and the Underdogs—Harvey Mason Jr. and Damon Thomas. The Underdogs had produced all of my tracks from the *Dreamgirls* album, so I was extremely comfortable working with them. They knew me really well, so it helped to have that rapport in the studio. And since I was signed with Clive, no one in the music business was out of reach. I even had the chance to work with the legendary Jimmy Jam and Terry Lewis, who became teachers to me. Terry became a father figure, too. He always had a life lesson to share, and I was always willing to listen. I practically lived in their Los Angeles studio while we worked on our songs together. Unfortunately, none of those songs ended up on the final album, but I will never forget the relationships that were formed as a result.

had been traveling around the country with David that summer, promoting the upcoming release of my album. Since I had booked a show in Boston, David was excited to take me on a tour of Harvard, where he attended law school. I loved seeing college through his eyes and sharing in his history prior to meeting me. Our relationship was growing.

was floored and honored that I was asked to sing the national anthem for the opening of the Democratic National Convention, held in Denver on August 25, 2008. I knew it was going to be a defining moment in our country's history, but I had no idea how impactful that experience would be for me. I sang for all of the constituents and politicians in attendance, including the new Democratic presidential nominee, Barack Obama. Being from the same hometown, it was truly a thrill to sing for him. As with so many events I am privileged to be a part of, I could hardly believe that I had been given the opportunity to be a part of this historic occasion. Although my brother and sister weren't able to be with me, they kept calling to see how I was doing. My sister kept asking if I was nervous—which I wasn't. I was so excited to get out there and represent Chicago that I could hardly wait for my moment. My brother kept reminding me that the altitude in Denver might make me woozy or parched before I sang. Thank God he warned me because just before I was set to walk out onto the stage, I got so light-headed, I almost passed out. Thankfully, it was just the altitude, so I gave myself a minute or two to pull it together and was able to go out and sing with no problem.

David, my mama, and my aunt were also with me on this trip. Mama never liked being in the spotlight, but she sure loved to be with me at all of my important events. And I was so happy having her by my side. Unbeknownst to me, David used that opportunity to spend a few minutes alone with my mama to ask for her blessing in marriage. Thank God my mama said yes! According to David, he let out a big sigh of relief.

A couple of weeks later, David and I were in Los Angeles—our last stop of the many appearances I'd done to promote the upcoming album release. It was my twenty-seventh birthday.

David took me on a drive up the Pacific Coast Highway . . . and when he parked the car, he asked me to marry him. I was truly shocked. David had picked out the perfect ring for me! I was going to get married . . . someday. Of course, I started thinking about all the things girls think about when they get engaged. The date. The venue. The dress. Looking like a princess in the dress. But those wedding plans were going to have to wait. I had an album coming out, and David had big plans for his career that he wanted to pursue.

Shortly after David and I became engaged, David made a decision to pursue a passion of his that would ultimately change the course of his life and his career. David wanted to become a professional wrestler for the WWE. This was his dream, and when he was given the opportunity to turn that dream into a reality, he took it. The one glitch was that David would have to move to Tampa, Florida, to train for several months, which meant we were suddenly going to be in a long-distance relationship. But I wanted David to live his dream just like I was living mine. We figured out that I could come to Tampa on weekends, or whenever there was an opportunity, so we wouldn't go long periods without seeing each other. A week after being asked to join the WWE, David packed up and left for Tampa. My life was changing so fast.

My album finally dropped on September 27, 2008. I remember that day like it was yesterday. I was so excited but incredibly frightened, too. A lot was riding on the success of this record. As I said, you never get a second chance to make your first record. I always get nervous right before I go onstage. I am putting myself out there and trusting the audience will embrace whatever I have to give. Releasing an album is that same feeling—only on steroids. Even though I was a nervous wreck, I went down to my local record store the day the album came out so I could see it on the shelves for myself.

*This* was the moment I had waited for my entire life.

The album was simply called *Jennifer Hudson*. I figured the world that knew me as the actress who played Effie White needed to know me as the singer Jennifer Hudson. The cover was a simple black-and-white photo of me. I had recently cut my hair short and wore a dress the stylist picked out for me, with a wide belt at the waist.

Imagine my surprise when I saw the album cover. I had clearly been Photoshopped to look thinner for the cover of my record. I had not been told this was going to happen, and I was pretty shocked. So were my fans, and many of them voiced their disappointment since a lot of them had identified with me as a plus-size gal. It was another case of needing to fit an image. But I was able to put that disappointment aside for the excitement that came with finally having an album of my own, for the world to hear.

There were three singles from the album, including the first, "Spotlight," which was released as a single in June 2008 before the record dropped. The other two singles were "If This Isn't Love" and "Giving Myself," which were later released in 2009.

"Spotlight" was my first top-30 hit, peaking at number twenty-four on the Billboard Hot 100 and becoming a top-20 hit in the United Kingdom. The song peaked at number one on the Billboard Hot R&B/Hip-Hop Songs, spending two consecutive weeks in the top spot.

When I was a little girl, I used to dream about the day when I would make my own music video. Thank God I spent so much time rehearsing in the mirror as a kid because when it came time to actually do the video for "Spotlight," I was ready. Even though there was a music video for "And I Am Telling You I'm Not Going," it was just the scene from the movie. This was different because that video belonged to Effie—and "Spotlight" was all mine. The choreographer was shocked at how natural I appeared. He said I didn't look like an amateur. Of course not! I had prepared my whole life for this moment.

When I read the various treatments for the video, I wasn't really sure what to think. They wanted to put me in tight, sexy clothes and spiky high heels for a scene that had me "at home on the couch."

I remember thinking, Now, why would I have on heels? I hate wearing high heels! In fact, someday I want to find a way to create a sexy heel girls can walk in all day long without their feet getting sore. Can I please get an Amen on that?

We shot the video in a Los Angeles studio. I decided to bring my own clothes to the shoot. The process of shooting this video took a really long time. We ended up shooting until four a.m. the next day, and I had to stand in those high heels the whole time. By the last shot, my feet were killing me! Luckily, the video turned out well, and I was very happy with the final product and liked working with the director, Chris Robinson. Sore feet were a small price to pay.

The album did better than the label expected. The album made its debut on the Billboard 200 and the Top R&B/Hip-Hop Albums chart with first week's sales of 217,000 copies. It was eventually certified gold for selling more than a half million copies.

I n the fall of 2008, I had started a new weight-loss regimen in preparation for a film adaptation of Winnie Mandela's life called *Winnie*. I had been cast to play the amazing Winnie Mandela under the assumption that I would lose a significant amount of weight to look more like her. I noticed I was feeling unusually tired. I know my body, and something felt very different. I wasn't sure if the way I was feeling was due in part to my new dieting habits, stress, or perhaps some combination of both.

I didn't think I was pregnant because I had no obvious symptoms. Even so, I decided to take a home pregnancy test just to rule it out. I stood in the bathroom and waited for my results. I couldn't help but let my mind wander and think about the possibility . . . and the irony.

I looked down.

Positive.

I was pregnant.

The only person we decided to tell right away was my manager so that he could let the producers of *Winnie* know I wouldn't be able to do the movie anytime soon. We didn't give them an exact reason. We just told them it was personal. Thankfully, they agreed to wait it out because they didn't want to recast the lead. They wanted me to play Winnie and were willing to wait. The producers told me to do whatever I needed to do and that they would be ready whenever I was. I couldn't have asked for anything more. I thanked them for their gracious patience and understanding.

David and I loved to take weekend trips to amusement parks like Disney World and Universal Studios. I had always loved going on rides. One day we approached a ride that had a sign posted that read, "Do not ride this if you are pregnant." Funny, I had ridden this roller coaster many times before I was pregnant, but had never noticed that sign until that day. I stood there for a moment trying to figure out what to do. I couldn't make up my mind. The people behind us in line were getting annoyed for sure. Of course, no one knew I was pregnant so they couldn't understand my hesitation. These types of decisions were all so new and unfamiliar to me.

I suddenly went from thinking for myself to thinking like a mama in thirty seconds flat and have never looked back since. Going forward, everything I did, every decision I made, and every road traveled would be considered with my baby's welfare in mind first. It was exciting to approach life from this brand-new perspective, and even better, without anyone knowing why—at least for a little while.

I had been keeping a pretty low profile, but I couldn't stay out of the spotlight forever. I was asked to sing the national anthem at the 2009 Super Bowl, scheduled in Tampa on February 2. It was an easy decision since I didn't even have to fly anywhere. Thankfully, I wasn't showing yet, so I wasn't worried about anyone finding out that I was pregnant. Although I had been on one of the most-watched television shows on the planet, *American Idol*, I don't think there is a larger audience and platform than the Super Bowl. God gave me the nerves of steel that I needed that night. This was the first time I was stepping out since the tragedy that struck my family. It was a very strange evening because I had never been hounded or stalked by the media like I was that night. It was overwhelming. When I stood on the field facing the crowd, there was a roar in the stadium unlike anything I had ever heard. Luckily, once I started to sing, the tension faded away, as it always does. Singing is always my saving grace. I sang from my heart and soul that night—and I think it showed.

Even though we had been given a skybox to watch the game, as soon as I hit that last note, I was eager to leave. David stayed and watched the game with my brothers and a few other relatives while I headed straight from the stadium to the nearest Chipotle, in full hair and makeup. A pregnant woman wants what she wants!

The next time I would sing in public was at the 2009 Grammy Awards. I wore a black-and-white dress that strategically hid my ever-growing baby bump. I simply wasn't ready to let the world know I was expecting, much less answer questions from the press. That night, I worked with a new stylist who kept trying to put me into undergarments that were way too tight across my belly. I had to tell her I wouldn't wear them. I also had to tell her not to push on my stomach, but I never told her why. Hopefully she only thought I was just strangely obsessed with my abs. At my record label, no one ever suggested that I might be pregnant, though I wonder if they suspected. No one ever asked me. And really, when you think about it, who asks a grown woman if she's pregnant, anyway? What if she isn't? Boy, that's awkward.

The Grammys that year were pretty special to me, wardrobe

issues or not. My album received three nominations, including Best Female R&B Vocal Performance for "Spotlight," Best R&B Performance by a Duo or a Group with Vocal for "I'm His Only Woman," a duet I recorded with Fantasia Barrino, and Best R&B Album, for which I ended up winning the award.

Winning a Grammy was a dream come true for two very special reasons. To begin with, it was my first, and a great vote of confidence in my music career from my peers. And while that *was* truly exciting, receiving that award from Whitney Houston, my idol and greatest musical influence, was the icing on the cake. I couldn't believe I was standing right next to her on the same stage, much less receiving an award from her. I was in complete awe, but not for the first time when it came to Ms. Whitney Houston.

I actually met Whitney Houston for the first time at a charity event in October 2006. It was one of the first times in my life that I can honestly say I was starstruck. I was scheduled to sing during the event and was sitting in a hallway inside the Beverly Hilton hotel, where the fund-raiser was taking place. I was waiting to go into the ballroom to perform. My publicist and choreographer were sitting with me when I noticed a herd of men rushing down the hallway looking like secret service. They were surrounding a woman and walking very fast. When I looked up, I realized it was Whitney. As she passed by us, she held up her index finger and said, "Stop."

Her entourage stopped cold in their tracks.

Whitney walked over to me and stood about three inches from my face.

"You. You're the one." She practically whispered when she spoke.

I had no idea what she was talking about. I was mesmerized and frozen by her presence. It was such a surprise that Whitney Houston came over . . . to me!

"You're the one. It is you. I know you."

My publicist elbowed me to get up out of my seat, but I couldn't move. Before I could say anything, she was gone.

I didn't see Whitney Houston again until the night of the Grammys. If there was anything that could have lifted my spirits at this time, it was receiving my first Grammy Award from her. As a way of showing my appreciation and respect for everyone who had reached out to me over the months since the family tragedy I had just endured, for my Grammy performance I chose to sing a song from my album called "You Pulled Me Through." When I recorded the song, I had no idea why I was singing it, but I knew it had a purpose. Singing it that night helped me discover that purpose. That song suddenly made perfect sense because I felt as if I had seen the highest of the highs and the lowest of the lows in my life. Rickey Minor, my musical director at the time, told me that I am a storyteller and I could paint the picture for an audience through my music. I knew that song had the potential to reach people on a deeply spiritual level—and in the end, I believe it did.

If it's true that God never gives us anything more than we can handle, he sure knew I would be able to handle things that night. I was able to go out there and still have a sweet taste in my mouth after all of the bitterness I had suffered. I've always been emotional when I sing, but on this particular night I was extremely so. As I've said, my crying through a song used to irritate my mama. She'd say, "Jenny, why do you have to be crying when you're up there to sing. What are you crying for, baby girl?" On that night, I was thinking of my family and just wanted to make them proud. I didn't care if I cried or not. I don't think anyone did.

I don't think there was a dry eye in the house.

After the Grammys, I agreed to perform on *American Idol* for the first time since I was voted off. I have to admit, it felt good to be back on that stage. It was like going home. For sure I thought someone there would notice my belly—but they didn't! I even appeared on *The Oprah Winfrey Show* and *The Ellen DeGeneres Show* around this time, and even though I was now several months pregnant, no one ever said a word.

I tried maintaining my regular diet and exercise routine for the first four months of the pregnancy. My first trimester was easy. I had no signs or symptoms that I was carrying a baby and therefore often forgot that I was. David was terrified as I'd race up flights of stairs, go for a run, or do anything physical. I felt great and kept living my life as I normally did. Funny things started to happen though, like not being able to stand the smell of David's cologne and an occasional unexplained meltdown over the smallest things. I never wore maternity clothes throughout my pregnancy. I just wore my regular clothes, though I went for the looser stretchy ones as my belly grew. This was a big realization for me . . . maybe I did need to think about losing some weight after this baby was born. If I could wear my regular clothes during pregnancy, maybe they were a little . . . big.

By my fifth month, my hormones really took over and my body wanted me to eat whatever it wanted to eat. I like spicy food and was craving it morning, noon, and night. I remember going to a Mexican restaurant to order up some nachos (without onions, of course) to go. I was very specific about what I did and did not want on my nachos. The waitress took my order just as I had given it— *no* onions! Unfortunately, when I opened the box in the car, those nachos were covered in everything I had asked them to skip. I was so mad that I threw them out the window! Now, maybe it was the hormones that caused me to act that way—but everyone knows you don't play with a pregnant woman's food!

As he always did, David acted nonchalant about the scene I had just caused. Looking back, I hope it wasn't because I had been acting that way so often he was no longer fazed by that behavior. Oh well. You *can* get away with more when you're pregnant, right, ladies?

Not long after this, my sister sent me a text that said, "If one more person asks me if you're pregnant, I'm going to give them a due date. Jenny—what's the deal?" she asked.

I texted her back with my due date, and that's how I told Julia I was pregnant.

I then wanted to make sure my whole family knew the good news now, before the press started talking. So in the spring of 2009, I decided it was time to make an official announcement to my big family. It had been a while since I had seen them. As I said, I was still wearing my regular clothes, so even after I shared the good news, everyone thought I was playing a trick on them. My aunts were all there that day, and in my family, all I really needed to do was tell my aunts. Sure enough, shortly afterward, everyone else in the extended family was finally in the know.

The rest of the world found out I was pregnant when I sang at Michael Jackson's memorial on July 7, 2009. The service was held at the Staples Center and was covered by the media worldwide. By this time I was eight months pregnant and really only wanted to be at home resting. I was getting uncomfortable and just wanted my baby out and my body back. Of course, Michael's death was so sudden and unexpected. So I was happy to be part of the celebration of his life and to have my chance to honor Michael. It was a sad but amazing day, and I was glad that I was included, despite feeling very tired at this point.

Even though my sister has special feelings about these things and had predicted that we were going to have a boy, David and I never knew the sex of our baby until he was born. We shopped for a boy and a girl and had outfits for both in my suitcase that I took to the hospital. We had names picked out for both, too. We had resigned ourselves that whatever it was going to be, it would be.

When the baby came, David said, "It's a boy, Jenny!"

I could hear my son yelling and screaming. He definitely inherited my strong voice!

And there he was—my little munchkin. David placed our baby atop my chest so I could feel his little heart beat against mine. He looked just like a mini version of David. We named him David Daniel Otunga Jr.

It was love at first sight.

As I held him close, I cried more than my newborn son.

My circle of life was now complete. I had a man I loved and, together, we brought a new life into the world. After everything we had been through, we were both so happy. I couldn't think of a better way to honor my mother than becoming a mother myself. From the very moment my son was born, I have felt my mama's presence guiding me. She was such a great role model in so many ways. I want to be that same kind of inspiration to my son, too. And now, I had the rest of my life to do just that.

I loved being a mom from the very start. Little David is the light of my life. Whenever I had to travel for work in those first few months, I did what I had to do and hurried back home to be with my son. I had someone waiting for me, someone who unconditionally loved me with all his heart, and someone I couldn't wait to hold in my arms. I cherish every moment we have together.

Munchkin quickly developed his own unique personality. The older he got, the more of me I saw in him. My son never met an audience he didn't like. He loves the sound of a cheering crowd. Maybe it is because I performed so much during my pregnancy, the sound of a clapping audience is familiar to him.

About a year or so after David Jr. was born, I was doing a show in Barbados. The crowd began to cheer in the middle of one of my songs. I thought it was odd, but chalked it up to the audience just feeling the music. I looked to my right and noticed Munchkin standing off in the corner of the stage with his own microphone in his hands. They were cheering for *him*—not me.

I asked my engineer to turn up the house lights so David could see the audience. He loved it. He had no fear whatsoever. As long as he is happy, I am, too. I guess we will all have to wait and see what happens!

# CHAPTER EIGHT

# I AM CHANGING

Within days of bringing David home from the hospital, I made a decision that ultimately altered my health for life. Becoming a mother brought on tremendous responsibilities, but none greater than the obligation I felt to get healthy to be there for my son.

I gained thirty-five pounds during my pregnancy. Like most women, I was shocked that even after giving birth, I still weighed around 237 pounds. I felt that surely I would drop at least some of the weight once that baby came out. This was the biggest number I had seen on the scale in many years. It was time to think about how I was going to lose the excess baby weight and then put that plan into action.

Since I had given birth via C-section, I was unable to do much of anything for the first ten days or so. I could barely get off the sofa and couldn't walk fully upright without pain for some time. For six weeks after giving birth, going to the gym or working out was definitely out of the question. What I could do during that time was try to break my body's cravings for the unhealthy foods I freely ate during the last few months of my pregnancy. While I didn't completely go crazy, I didn't deprive myself of anything while I was pregnant, either. If I wanted cupcakes—I ate them. If I wanted Mexican food—and I did often—I ate it. So when the time came to gain control over my eating again and hopefully once and for all, I fell back into my old diet mentality that had worked for me so many times before having my baby.

It was an all-too-familiar routine. I had grown comfortable with eating skinless baked chicken, brown rice, and steamed broccoli—morning, noon, and night. My staple diet foods. My big treat was two apple slices with peanut butter slathered on top. I only drank water and occasionally treated myself to Crystal Light. That way of eating is effective for quick weight loss, but it isn't very interesting. And like anything, if we get bored we change things up, and usually not in our favor. It's a total setup for failure because eating that way forever just isn't realistic.

Once I was finally able to get active, I started walking a loop around my neighborhood that took close to thirty minutes to complete. To be honest, when I first began taking these walks, this same route took me closer to an hour because I had to take it slow.

After a few weeks I was able to cut that time in half. I relished these walks by myself because those precious moments were my "thinking" time. I enjoy being outdoors, especially when it's really hot and humid. I put my headphones on and away I go. I do most everything with music playing in my ears. It gives me motivation to get up off that sofa and inspiration to take those extra laps. But sometimes, the motivation was hard to come by. If the baby had been up a lot or he was napping and I could get a few quiet moments at home, sometimes I just wanted to stay on the couch.

Whenever I'd try to talk myself out of going for a walk, and there were a few days like that, I'd take myself through a series of simple tasks so I would get up and go.

**1. Get up.**

**2. Find your house keys.**

**3. Put on some shoes.**

**4. Grab your iPod.**

**5. Walk out the front door.**

Like I said, I like to set goals for myself, and these small goals got me out the door more than a few times.

And if after all that I still didn't move from the chair, as a sure-fire way of talking myself into just doing it, I'd trick myself by saying, "It is okay to walk for just ten minutes—because that would be better than doing nothing." And once I got up, ten minutes turned into thirty and eventually an hour. It got to the point where I would begin to miss how good I felt from working out that I'd actually get inspired by that, too.

*According to the Organization for Economic Cooperation and Development (OECD), the number of obese people in the United States will increase from 99 million in 2008 to 164 million by 2030. The U.S. obesity rate will rise from 32 percent to about 50 percent for men and from 35 percent to between 45 percent and 52 percent for women.*

Later in the year, when I was well on my way to losing the baby weight I had gained, I met with a team of people from Weight Watchers. They sat with me and explained the principles of their program. The best way to think about the program is as a plan that gives its members a personalized budget of Points values per day. Your available Points are calculated based on your weight, age, and activity level. Every food has a Points value and you use those values to fill your day up with food. You keep track of your Points by writing down everything you eat. There is flexibility in the program in this regard, but many members cite tracking what they eat and the values associated with their food as the key to their success.

To be frank, I thought it all sounded lame and I wasn't all that interested. All I could think of was, Who wants to eat and then have to write all of that down? I was polite, but I felt like this program was in no way right for me.

The representative said that the way the numbers work is that they quantify food for you. They show you that one food choice is better than another based on the Points assigned to that food. For example, a processed nutrition bar, which is something most people think of as a good choice when trying to lose weight, might have a seven *PointsPlus*® value and may carry as many as two hundred and fifty calories. On the other hand, a banana has a zero *PointsPlus*® value and will actually keep you fuller for longer than a protein bar. It has more fiber and more water and vitamins, too. So the program quantifies food in a way that teaches you to navigate the environment that we all live in. As I listened, one of the more promising aspects of the program for me was learning that the program builds in some extra flexibility for you because they know that if you don't get in some of the things you love—the sweets you crave and such—you won't stick with the plan. They actually give you an added allowance of an extra forty-nine Points every week so you can have those things along the way.

What this means is, if you're going to a wedding over the weekend and you don't want to sit it out because you're afraid of breaking the plan, you can still go. You can even have a cocktail or a piece of the wedding cake without worrying about your Points allowance for the day. If a friend calls you to go to dinner and you've already had twenty-five of your daily twenty-nine Points, you can pull from the extra forty-nine allowed for the week. It gives a kind of real-life flexibility I had never seen in any other plan. When I first talked to Weight Watchers, they hadn't yet launched their current program, *PointsPlus*®, but did so soon after. It is now in full swing and has been used by millions to great results.

## About the Weight Watchers® *PointsPlus*® Program

The biggest innovation from Weight Watchers in more than a decade, *PointsPlus*® uses the latest scientific research to create a program that goes far beyond traditional calorie counting to give people the edge they need to lose weight and keep it off in a fundamentally healthier way.

The program is designed to educate and encourage people to make choices that:

- Favor foods the body works harder to convert into energy, resulting in fewer net calories absorbed.

- Focus on foods that create a sense of fullness and satisfaction and are more healthful.

- Nudge toward natural foods rather than foods with excess added sugars and fats.

- Still allow flexibility for indulgences, special occasions, and eating out.

## HOW IT WORKS

While calorie counting has been the foundation of many weight-loss programs, including the Weight Watchers former *Points®* system, the *PointsPlus®* program goes beyond just calories to help people make healthful and satisfying choices.

The formula takes into account the energy contained in each of the components that make up calories—protein, carbohydrates, fat, and fiber—and it also factors in how hard the body works to process them (conversion cost) as well as their respective eating satisfaction (satiety). As a result, the *PointsPlus®* formula guides people beyond reducing overall calorie intake toward foods that enhance feelings of satisfaction and fullness.

In addition to the new formula, foods that are low in energy density, and therefore more highly satisfying, are emphasized within the program. Specifically, all fresh fruits and most vegetables now have zero *PointsPlus®* values. Furthermore, power foods, an important element of the new *PointsPlus®* program, provide an easy way to identify the best food choices among similar foods; for example, those foods with higher eating satisfaction, lower sugar, lower sodium, healthier fat, and more fiber, and it also factors how hard the body works to process them (conversion cost) as well as their respective eating satisfaction (satiety). As a result, the *PointsPlus®* formula guides people beyond reducing overall calorie intake toward foods that enhance feelings of satisfaction and fullness.

The program features, combined with the fundamentals of the Weight Watchers approach—that is, weight loss built on healthy eating, physical activity, behavior modification, and a supportive environment—make the *PointsPlus®* program revolutionary and innovative.

## PROGRAM HIGHLIGHTS

*PointsPlus®* values reflect the energy that's available after the body has processed a food.

Power foods are an easy way to identify the best food choices among similar foods; for example, those foods with higher eating satisfaction, lower sugar, lower sodium, healthier fat, and more fiber.

Zero *PointsPlus*® values are assigned to fresh fruit and most vegetables, which are nutrient dense and are highly satisfying.

Weekly *PointsPlus*® gives an allowance of 49 extra *PointsPlus*® values per week, in addition to the daily *PointsPlus*® target. This allows for flexibility so members and online subscribers can avoid feeling deprived and are therefore motivated to stick with the program since real life often means unplanned eating opportunities.

Activity *PointsPlus*® values are used to reward activity because it is important for good health and is a critical component of weight loss. Members and online subscribers can track activity *PointsPlus*® values for motivation or they can swap them for extra food *PointsPlus*® values.

## INDUSTRY-LEADING RESEARCH AND PROVEN EFFECTIVENESS

The *PointsPlus*® program has been tested in a rigorous, independent clinical trial, and the results demonstrate that it delivers significant weight loss as well as improvements in decreasing cardiovascular risk factors and eating behaviors linked with long-term weight loss and hedonistic hunger.

The testing applied to this new program is a reflection of Weight Watchers' commitment to clinical testing with more than sixty-five original scientific publications over the past fifteen years that demonstrate the efficacy of the Weight Watchers approach to weight loss and long-term health.

Thousands of people across the United States were involved in beta testing the *PointsPlus®* program. In addition to being thrilled with their weight loss, these individuals reported they felt healthier and more satisfied. People shifted their choices away from energy-dense, processed foods toward fruit, vegetables, whole grains, and lean proteins, changing their life in a meaningful and natural way and demonstrating the effectiveness of the *PointsPlus®* program.

A global study recently published in *The Lancet* indicated that overweight and obese adults referred to Weight Watchers lost more than twice as much weight when compared with those who received standard care. This study provides significant evidence to the value of a primary care and Weight Watchers partnership for an effective weight-loss approach.

I listened carefully as the folks from Weight Watchers explained the program, but I still didn't believe most of what they were saying. I nodded in agreement, but they lost me at "You can eat whatever you want."

I thought, There is no way I can eat those types of foods and lose weight, because it was against everything I knew about weight loss and healthy eating. My mind was programmed to think deprivation, not freedom of choice. No one can sustain a diet of grilled skinless chicken, brown rice, and steamed broccoli forever. Eventually you have to nourish your body with something else, and when you do, the weight comes right back. I would stop myself from having the foods I loved until the cravings got so bad I couldn't take it for one more second. I'd inevitably break down and give in by heading to my favorite chicken wing place, ordering a huge box of wings, and eating the entire thing. Afterward, I'd feel so bad about making that choice, the next day I'd go right back on my extreme deprivation diet until I'd repeat the same pattern over and over again.

I had been so brainwashed into believing that dieting meant excruciating limitations that I had rejected the principles of the Weight Watchers program. I simply didn't believe I could eat chips, cookies, or pizza and lose weight. My mind was made up. There was no way their plan would work. But out of courtesy, I reluctantly agreed to try the program for one week.

Weight Watchers assigned a woman named Liz Josefsberg to be

my Weight Watchers leader. Liz was there to help me understand and then navigate my plan on the program. The first thing Liz and I spoke about was the ways I'd lost weight before and what I had done to take off the excess baby weight. She recognized that I had what she called "a lot of diet baggage" left over from my past.

By the time I met Liz, I had lost a fair amount of weight on my own, but as it usually did, my weight hit the familiar plateau around 193 pounds. It seemed that no matter what I tried, I couldn't break through. Liz spent a great deal of time talking to me about small healthy changes I could make that would get me there.

Although I was already a pretty healthy eater for the most part, and had a lot of firsthand knowledge about losing weight, Liz helped me see that I was making tiny mistakes that were throwing me off and keeping my weight loss stagnant. For example, I knew I was eating good snack choices, such as trail mix with nuts and dried fruit. What I didn't realize was the amount I was eating was actually detrimental. Liz asked me how much trail mix I'd eat in a sitting and the truth is, I didn't know. I ate my snack without paying any attention to the amount. I was aware that I was eating several handfuls at a time—if not more—but I had no idea how much that really added up to. Liz suggested trying a quarter cup at a sitting instead of eating as much as I wanted. That seemed reasonable enough, although at the time, I wasn't sure what a quarter of a cup actually looked like. I shared with Liz that I also loved eating Greek yogurt with peanut butter. Once again, Liz asked me how much peanut butter I was eating with that serving of yogurt.

Again, I didn't know.

She explained that one tablespoon of peanut butter is a great choice for a snack, but adding a giant dollop into the yogurt can throw me out of my weight-loss zone. When Liz pointed out that the food choice was right but the amount was the problem, I realized that *portion control* and *lack of awareness* were my two biggest challenges to weight loss.

Liz gave me a visual demonstration on what amounts of food were doable in the Weight Watchers program and what amounts would set me back. Next, she reintroduced me to all the foods I could eat—as long as they were measured in the right amounts. It was interesting to see, but the fact remained that I was still in my "diet" mentality, so I thought she was crazy as she told me that I could have ice cream, chocolate, popcorn, pizza, and sushi. Sushi! It's one of my most favorite meals on the planet and I hadn't eaten it for two years because of the high carbohydrates in the rice and because I was avoiding it while pregnant. The promise was enticing, but the reality seemed a little suspect.

"What do I do when I get a craving for chicken wings?" I asked, knowing damn well those would never be a choice on a healthy weight-loss program.

"You can eat wings, but eat six instead of twelve. Have a green salad first so you're not as hungry by the time you get to the wings," Liz said. "If you don't branch outside of what you know, you will break down, which means you will fall away from the program, and we don't want that to happen."

Hold on.

She was insistent that I could eat whatever I wanted and all I had to do was track the Points and I would lose weight?

Was she serious?

She was. For the first time ever, that was exactly what someone was telling me. I could not believe it, so I did what I always do when I can't wrap my brain around an idea.

I said, "Whatever."

Uh-huh. I did. I said it. I said, "Whatever," and by now we all know how that movie ends.

Sensing my doubt, Liz insisted that as long as I stayed within my allotted-Points-per-day budget, I would definitely lose weight. At the end of the day, the Weight Watchers program is an education in sidestepping the misinformation out there about dieting, and breaking the negative diet mentality that predominates the world we all live in. Weight Watchers hands you the tools to make the right choices. But you still have to make those choices or the program, like any program, won't work.

I found that out the hard way.

I still had my doubts, but as I said, out of courtesy I agreed to give Weight Watchers a try. I figured I would give it a week to see what happened. Honestly, I had nothing to lose—except a few pounds. But of course, I wasn't expecting that to happen. If I wasn't satisfied with the results, then I could just as easily go back to my old way of dieting. Nothing ventured, nothing gained.

The first week on the program I created my own version of the Weight Watchers program. I mostly stuck to what I had already been doing and combined it with some of the food choices Liz said I could have. Nice try, but I didn't lose a pound. It turned out that Jenny Kate's way didn't quite meet the criteria set for me by Weight Watchers. When I saw Liz a week later, she wasn't shocked by my lack of results, because she immediately knew I hadn't stuck with the program. Then Liz shared that I was like a lot of her other members. I didn't *trust* the program. She was absolutely right about that.

By the second week, I had actually gained weight. I think I tried that first week five different times before I realized I had two roads I could walk down on this journey. I could keep doing things my way and keep getting the same dismal results, or I could finally give in and try Weight Watchers for real, and see what happened.

I decided to give the plan a try. I fully committed. Here's what I discovered: Weight Watchers is not a painful program. I was like most people, believing that weight loss has to be a struggle and a painful experience. It *can* be that, but it doesn't have to be. Through Weight Watchers, you can learn to take weight off in a healthy manner without giving up all the foods that make you feel good. After my first real week, I lost five pounds. With that result, I actually wanted to stick to their program.

"Walter! I don't know what they did, but this plan works!" I was excited by my progress. I thought I had found the weight-loss miracle. "This is it. This is all I need." From that moment on, I was hooked. "You got me," I said to Liz. And they did. I even agreed to sign on as a spokeswoman for the company—an ambassador of sorts—and I haven't looked back since.

My contract to be an ambassador for Weight Watchers only called for me to lose 10 percent of my body weight. That's it. No more, no less. Needless to say, that goal was met pretty early on. After that, I didn't stick with the plan out of some contractual obligation. No way. It became a healthy lifestyle choice for me—one that helped me discover a program that was not only doable but also realistic for sustained weight loss.

My relationship with Liz became one of the most important in my journey to regain my health. I connected with her from the start. She was easy to talk to and understood me from the beginning. When we first met, Liz explained that all Weight Watchers leaders were once members, and to become a leader, she had to have been on the program. Knowing that helped me because she could relate to everything I was going through. Liz told me that before joining the company, she had lost and gained the same thirty pounds several times over the years. Frustrated after many failed diets, she decided to join Weight Watchers as her last hope. She eventually lost fifty pounds and has kept it off, which gave me a tremendous amount of comfort and confidence in her. She knew what it was like to lose that much weight, so I could really open up to her along the way. Liz knew where I was coming from and was able to answer all my questions, and address my concerns and challenges as we forged ahead.

I was lucky to have the relationship I developed with Liz, but it's important to know that my experience was very much like anyone who is a member of the program. Every Weight Watchers meeting has a leader there to support you through your own journey. And while your schedule and challenges may not be the same as mine, we are all busy just living our lives—doing the best we can. I can promise you that if you trust in the program and trust your leader, you will see positive results. In doing my own research, there was no other plan out there that offered the healthy Weight Watchers message or support and, more so, delivered with the results.

# CHAPTER NINE

# FEELING GOOD

I t's important to me that you all know that the hard work I've done to take control of my health, I have done completely on my own. I don't live in a mansion with a private chef or personal trainer at my beck and call. Oh no. I get so frustrated when people make that imaginary leap that I live like a princess in a castle with all of my needs met by others. I cook my own meals, and when I can't because I'm on a movie set all day or in the recording studio, Walter takes care of making sure my meals are fixed as if I made them myself.

Whenever people ask me how they can lose weight, too, the first thing I tell them is that they have to make up their mind that they really want to do it and do it for themselves. I suppose that way of thinking is true for breaking any addiction, but for me, that was the difference in losing the weight and keeping it off. *If you can't take responsibility for your own well-being, you will never take control over it.* That is the truth.

Look, change is scary. If you aren't completely ready to make adjustments that will ultimately alter the course of your life, you are not ready to embrace change. My fiancé is the type of man who likes things to be the way they've always been. He doesn't like change, but he's been very supportive. He understands I did this for me and for me alone. You can't make a life-altering decision for someone else and expect it to stick. Gaining control over your health and well-being is one of those times in your life that you get to be completely selfish and not feel bad about it. If you want to meet your goals, you have to make it about you. You have to make it work for you and you alone. Anything less is a setup for failure.

Listen, I have been through this weight-loss roller coaster a few times over the years. I have been there and back and there and back again and again. I had everyone on the planet tell me that I needed to look a certain way or be a specific size if I wanted to make it as a singer. I have been rejected from more jobs than the ones I've gotten simply because of my appearance. If I had listened to all of those people, maybe I would have become a broken-down, overweight, out-of-work, *American Idol* castoff has-been. But I didn't. I was never that insecure. I'm telling you the absolute truth when I say that I genuinely loved my body—fat, thin, and everywhere in between. If I didn't have that confidence, though, I don't think I could have forged ahead and continued to pursue my dreams. Loving yourself means caring enough to make the hard decisions in your life.

I have a friend who is a personal fitness trainer. One day he came to me to say he was getting fed up with a client of his because she wouldn't listen to him to get to a certain weight. We got to talking and I asked him if that number was what he wanted for her or what she wanted for herself. My friend looked at me like I had solved one of life's great mysteries. All this time, he was imposing what he wanted on his client without ever asking her what her goals were. Forget what everyone else wants you to do and figure out what you want for yourself. Here's what I know for sure: The only way you can sustain a permanent change is to create a new way of thinking, acting, and being.

When I decided to become an ambassador for Weight Watchers, I was ready to do whatever it took to get healthy and learn how to finally stay that way. My goals were to feel good, have enough energy and stamina to keep up with my son, get healthy, and not worry about my dress size anymore. And even though I was losing the weight for me, I had the greatest motivation on the planet—my brand-new baby son. Once I welcomed Munchkin into the world, I felt that I had an obligation to be the best mom I could be for him. He deserved to have a mama who could run after him, chasing him around the house without getting winded or tired. I wanted him to have a role model who could teach him to make healthy food choices along the way so he would have the right tools as he went through life. I needed him to grow up with a mama who always would be there for him by caring enough about herself to take control of her health and eating. Everything changed on the day he was born. And now, I had a partner in Weight Watchers to help me get to my goal, for life.

The program is designed so that members can expect a one- to two-pound drop in weight per week when following the program. Of course, there can be some fluctuation in terms of the amount of weight you may lose, especially in the beginning. You tend to lose a bit more during the first couple of weeks due to mostly losses in fluid. One of the biggest challenges to continued weight loss I had was planning my meals around my very full schedule. Liz helped me to take a look at a typical week for me and see where I was making my mistakes.

Was I missing meals?

Was I overeating?

Was I starving and then bingeing?

I now knew I was making mistakes in terms of volume, so that took some time to understand and fix. Since my eating is often sporadic and done on the fly, it was important to come up with meals that were filling and able to hold me over long periods of time. It is not unreasonable for me to go eight, ten, or even twelve hours in between meals, especially when I am on a movie set or in the studio recording. While I once thought that was desirable, through Weight

Watchers I learned it was actually hurting me. So when I did sit down to eat, the question that kept coming up was, "Where and how can I make this meal better for me?" I asked myself that question before every meal—especially in the beginning.

Better awareness became a project and an exercise in discipline that I created for myself so I could study my eating habits—good and bad. Doing this forced me to evaluate what I was about to put into my body. It also gave me the chance to check my *PointsPlus*® so I could make sure I wasn't using up the bulk of my daily allowance in one meal. It eventually helped me learn to use my Points wisely, something that really made a difference in my weight loss.

The real secret to my success on Weight Watchers was tracking my *PointsPlus*® values. I am super-strict about tracking every little thing I eat. Weight Watchers made it really easy for me to stick with the program because everything you need is available online. I even downloaded their application onto my iPhone so I can easily keep track of my Points all day long, no matter where I am. I never skip logging something in because I am only fooling myself if I don't keep track. I want to know exactly where I am with my Points throughout the day so I can budget them wisely for future meals. I've gotten so disciplined that I can now tally my *PointsPlus*® values in my head. After a while, I began to memorize specific *Points-Plus*® values for the foods I regularly ate. Even so, I still use the Weight Watchers tracking system every day to keep me on the right path. If you consistently do that, you cannot fail on this program.

Although it is a fairly new passion of mine, I discovered that I actually like cooking my own food. So throughout the program, I didn't eat any prepackaged foods of any kind. Although Weight Watchers makes a variety of food products, the *PointsPlus®* plan doesn't require you to eat them. It is all about real food in the real world. My goal was to learn to pick foods that were healthy choices, and since I travel a lot, they had to be readily available most anywhere I go. Although I resisted the notion at first, I eventually learned that it was desirable to have a certain amount of carbohydrates because they're fuel for your body. I also began eating more fiber because it helps move things out, if you know what I mean. I also discovered the importance of cutting back on salt and sugar. When I was a little girl, salt was a food group to me. I used to put salt on everything, including my ice cream. (Don't knock it until you've tried it! Salted caramel is a little bit of heaven!)

Eating a diet filled with added sugar, unhealthy fats, and refined grains can make it easy to gain weight and at the same time not get the necessary vitamins, minerals, and other nutrients that you need for good health. These foods are also not as filling and satisfying as nutritious foods like fruits and vegetables. I never thought about any of these things before starting Weight Watchers, but they can have an impact on the scale and are equally important to maintaining good health. Weight Watchers does a great job of teaching their members these valuable lessons through their literature, on their Web site, and in the meetings.

A funny thing happened on the way to losing my eighty pounds. Foods that used to taste good to me no longer do. For example, if I take a sip of a regular soda now, all I can taste is the sugar. I also learned that processed food tastes better because it contains a lot of artificial ingredients that are unnecessary. Foods that contain a lot of artificial flavors often include a lot of fat, sugar, or salt to increase the enjoyment of that food, but they are not filling, and no longer part of my diet.

Since I've lost all of my weight, people always want to know what I eat. Here's the amazing thing about the Weight Watchers plan—you can eat what you've always eaten as long as you are eating the right portion amounts. While I don't have a set weekly menu, I do have some favorites that have helped me get to my goal.

A typical breakfast for me became one of three meals: grilled chicken breast fajitas with brown rice, an egg-white omelet with smoked salmon, or a chicken and vegetable omelet. If I am feeling it, I might add some cheese to the eggs, but otherwise, I go without. It is critically important to measure out the right portions or you will make the common error of eating the right foods in the wrong amounts. I make sure to use only a half to a full cup of chicken per serving, which ranges from two to four Points on the plan, depending on how hungry I am. Once I learned about the dangers of eating too much salt, I stopped adding salt to my omelets, especially the smoked salmon omelet because there is already enough salt in the fish. If I am especially hungry that morning, I might add some

Weight Watchers plain no-fat yogurt and twelve smoked almonds to my menu, too. The Weight Watchers yogurt is one of the only prepackaged foods I eat. I really like the flavor and texture of their yogurt, and unlike other brands, theirs is low in sugar. I highly recommend it as an excellent addition to any meal.

If I don't eat the yogurt with my breakfast, I will usually make it my midmorning snack. I don't believe in wasting my Points on things like juice, which I consider to be nothing but extra sugar and empty calories. The only time I will drink a glass of orange juice is if I feel like my body is craving the vitamin C and there is nothing else available to satisfy that desire. Otherwise, I know I am going to be hungry later in the day and would rather use those two to six Points on something that will fill me up and sustain me a lot longer than a glass of OJ. Instead, I will choose to drink water, Crystal Light, or occasionally, a Diet Coke.

Another secret to my weight loss was learning to make lunch my biggest meal of the day. One of my favorite choices is a turkey burger. I love them, especially the turkey burgers from the Cheesecake Factory. The problem, though, is their portions are ridiculously huge, so when I order one, I eat only half. And believe me, that's plenty!

I get so frustrated with restaurants that make it hard for a person who wants to make the healthy choice by over-serving its portions. The temptation is often too great to stay strong, so most people will overeat. When it comes to intake, there really needs to be a sense of "too much of a good thing." Even a turkey burger can throw your entire Points for the day off if the serving size is for four instead of one. This becomes a slippery slope when eating out, especially when you order a salad thinking it is the healthier choice but because of the excessive amounts of salad dressing, that salad can contain as many as fifteen hundred calories or more!

Looking at a menu through Weight Watchers' eyes changed my entire perspective on eating out. The Weight Watchers program allows me to eat at any restaurant. One of my favorites now is a chain called Texas de Brazil. They not only offer a buffet of food but also serve you selections at the table. They offer everything from steak to sushi, and black beans, rice with gravy, and so much more. David and I used to eat there before I started Weight Watchers, and I hated going because I didn't think there was anything on the menu I could eat. I don't eat steak, so we mostly went there because David liked it. However, once I got acquainted with the dos and don'ts of the Weight Watchers program, I discovered there were lots of options for me on their menu.

Since I eat mostly chicken, turkey, and fish, what I discovered was that most restaurants are happy to accommodate special requests for how you want your food prepared. These days, I have no issue telling my server that I want my chicken grilled with no sauce, my fish broiled with no butter, and my vegetables steamed instead of sautéed. It's so easy once you know how to make the right choices. And believe it or not, it is still delicious!

Dinner varies for me because it depends on how many Points I have left at the end of my day. My favorite home-cooked meal is one of my childhood favorites. My mama used to make the most delicious turkey wings with roasted sweet potato fries or mashed sweet potatoes. Eating that meal reminds me of my mama's and grandma's houses growing up. It smells like home to me. I don't eat a lot of fried foods, but I still like my turkey to crunch, so I boil the wings and then I put them in the oven where they can get as crispy as they can. I then take the juice from the bottom of the pan and sauté some greens in it to go as a side dish. Now this is some good old-fashioned home-style cooking!

Naturally, I can't eat like that all the time, so another favorite dinner dish is salmon. I was fixing dinner for David one night when I accidentally grabbed cinnamon instead of paprika to put on the fish. I didn't realize my mistake until we sat down to eat. It turned out to be so good that now, I *only* use cinnamon and lemon when I cook salmon. The cinnamon with lemon creates a glazelike finish on the fish that's a little like sweet teriyaki with no sugar. David loves it and I feel like I've got my B. Smith on when I make this dish for him.

Let me be really honest. I can get extremely bored eating the same old things over and over. It has always been one of my biggest pitfalls in dieting. My old cycle was to break my routine by eating something that wasn't a good choice. Now I've learned that I can change things up by getting creative with my meals and snacks. The Weight Watchers Web site offers thousands of meal ideas, recipes, and even snack options from other members. Snacks are an important part of the Weight Watchers plan, because working healthy snacks into your day means that you keep your hunger in check and don't overdo it at mealtime. One snack I love is almonds, and they are a really good healthy snack choice. On the Weight Watchers plan, they don't have a high *PointsPlus*® value, so I often turn to almonds as a favorite treat. When I am in the mood for something salty and crunchy, I will eat smoked almonds to satisfy my salt craving in a healthy way.

When it comes to making choices for my snacks, my general rule of thumb is to go for the real thing over an imitation. I especially love mixed fruit and melon. If I want orange sherbet, I'll reach for an orange instead of the ice cream. It's the flavor I'm going for so why not eat something that has fiber and nutrients over something that is full of chemicals and artificial flavors?

Okay, so here's the money question everyone always wants to know about.

Do I eat dessert?

The answer is . . . yes!

I have a terrible weakness when it comes to chocolate and banana pudding. I especially love Walter's banana pudding. When I was living in Miami and recording, I was in the studio most of the time. And when I wasn't, I was running along the beach and exercising in the gym. I thought I was staying on top of my weight until my stylist came to fit me for the MTV Video Music Awards. Not one single thing fit. I was so mad, thinking she just brought all the wrong sizes. No, it wasn't that. You see, Walter was making banana pudding all the time back then. I had tasted it way too much. I put a banana pudding moratorium in place right away. I told Walter he was no longer allowed to come into my house with that evil pudding. My biggest lesson there was that you cannot just work out and then eat poorly and expect to lose weight. It doesn't work that way.

One of the tools Weight Watchers taught me to become consciously aware of what I was eating and when, was to keep a journal and write down everything I ate and how I was feeling at the moment of making a decision. Liz explained that doing this would help me understand my triggers that create a habit. Weight Watchers was as much about building awareness as it was losing weight. The program makes you fully conscious of the food you put into your mouth and helps you to find a balance for everyday real life. Even though the program itself was astonishing in its results, it was this newfound awareness that became the game-changer for me.

Every person has to make the decision that they are ready to create awareness about what they are putting into their bodies and then work at learning to control that choice. For me, tuning in meant I began noticing that whenever I was home alone with

Munchkin, or worse, on my own, I often found myself hitting the refrigerator and then sitting on the sofa mindlessly eating. I was often very tired from staying up at night with the baby and wasn't always thinking about what I was eating so much as just eating. I discovered that I was especially vulnerable toward the end of my day, when I don't have any Points left without going into my reserve. One thing I often went for was chocolate. When I am relaxed and comfortable, I grab for some chocolate. I developed an obsession for chocolate bars when I was filming *Winnie* in Africa. To me, eating a piece of chocolate is as relaxing as a massage. It's an event. And when I am eating it, nobody better bother me because that is my moment of bliss. Some people like to have a glass of wine at the end of a busy day.

Me?

I like to eat some delicious chocolate.

Writing these habits down helped me pinpoint my weaknesses and become conscious of my behavior. With that awareness, I learned to make better choices. Instead of sitting on the sofa, I got up and exercised to a DVD. Or, if Munchkin was napping, I took a nap, too. If I decided to eat something, I ate something healthy like a handful of cashews and a few slices of apple. Let me tell you— when you put those two ingredients together, it is as good as a caramel apple—for real. And if I was going to have chocolate, I made sure it was really good chocolate, and in the right amount. Quality over quantity.

Another time I find it a challenge to make the right choices is when I am on a movie set. When I was making *The Three Stooges,* I really struggled with all of the sugary and salty foods that were kept out on the craft services table throughout the day. It was like that platter of cupcakes kept calling out my name. I decided the best way to combat that desire was to bring my own food from home and avoid the craft services table altogether. And when I couldn't stand it one second longer, I popped a piece of sugar-free gum into my mouth so I could have something sweet without grabbing for the pastries and such. Avoidance is a great tool to get away from food in my face all day long.

I learned to play little tricks on myself to avoid the trappings that used to keep a stronghold on me in the past. Pinkberry frozen yogurt used to be a passion of mine. Whenever I was in L.A., one of my first stops off the plane was Pinkberry to get a cup of their plain frozen yogurt with coconut, yogurt chips, and almonds sprinkled over the top. Now, instead of hitting Pinkberry when I land, I wait until the very end of my trip to treat myself so I won't have another opportunity to go back again before leaving town. That way I can't set myself up for failure or overdo a good thing. And I look forward to that Pinkberry all throughout my trip.

Even though I understood the benefits Liz was trying to share with me about journaling my feelings and hunger levels, it never really became my thing. Many people learn to use food for comfort or as a stress reliever. When they are angry, they like to chew on something crunchy or salty. Food is tied to emotion and is often used as an escape from those feelings. But I do know that for me, boredom was my biggest trigger. Even though I don't keep a journal, I do know this to be true for myself and I try to find ways to combat my boredom. What I learned from Weight Watchers is that food is meant to be used as fuel for our bodies. If we are using it for any other reasons, it is time to take a step back and ask ourselves what's up.

Once I was on the right path with the eating side of my quest for health, Liz helped me take a look at my exercise routines, too. Like my former diet mentality, my thought was that exercise had to be extreme to be effective. By this time, I had kicked up my exercise regimen to high-intensity training sessions several days a week that were leaving me sore and uncomfortable. I had adopted a "no pain, no gain" way of thinking, which left me mostly in pain with very little gain. Liz helped me realize that I could dial it back a bit and take it from being "work" to once again being enjoyable and fun. She did this by challenging me to stop doing things I didn't like and do only the things I enjoyed. That was a novel concept for me because even though I hadn't realized it for myself, somewhere along the way, exercise became a chore instead of a pleasure.

Although I always liked to exercise, at this time I had fallen into the extreme trap that took all of the fun out of it for me. The only real reward I was getting was the satisfaction of knowing that as long as I exercised hard, I could go out and eat whatever I wanted. Wrong! Liz explained that extreme exercise doesn't save you from poor food choices. It can be difficult to exercise and erase away that chocolate cake or pizza pie. It doesn't work that way. There is no such thing as a balanced equation with those things. If you're not eating the right foods in the right amounts, all the exercise in the world won't combat the caloric intake.

What was really hard to adjust to was that after I had my baby it became much harder to get out of the house to exercise. Even if I wanted to hit the gym, there were so many days I was too tired or tied to the house because Munchkin was sleeping. I started using that as an excuse not to do anything. Well, that didn't last long once I started the program.

Liz helped me embrace that the goal with exercise is to have as many options as possible. My close friends often call me "Random" because my workouts are never the same. I like doing fun things that I enjoy, from biking to basketball. Yeah, this sista's got game! I figure that as long as I am moving, I am burning calories. Some days I will choose to run outside or sprint up hills in our local park while others I'd rather use the treadmill at the gym. When I'm on the road, I still exercise to DVDs, especially when there isn't a gym available or when time is short. I like to run up and down stairs, too. I used to live on the twenty-sixth floor of my apartment building in Chicago and often took the stairs instead of taking the elevator. When your schedule is as busy as mine gets, you have to find windows of opportunity to do something active. Even if it's just going to and from the car—I'll take the harder, longer way to get there.

I'm a woman who likes progress. I want to see positive results for all of my efforts. If I am working out, then I expect to see a difference in my body. I'm definitely impatient, though. I hate waiting for anything, so the harder I work, the less time I need to wait to reap the rewards.

Like me, my fiancé is a workout fanatic, too. It's such a blessing to have a partner who shares your same beliefs in getting healthy as opposed to someone who is constantly trying to sabotage your efforts. David is a bodybuilder looking to bulk up his muscles and create mass while I am looking to slim down and elongate, so our workouts are completely different. When it comes to exercise, David never imposes his beliefs on me because we are going after two totally different looks.

The important message I heard about working out and what I want to share is that you create your own opportunities and your own limitations.

When I was assessing a diet plan that was right for me, I looked at many options—none of which made sense for my life. Every program I looked at was nothing more than a food plan. Either you are getting preprepared food delivered via the frozen-food section of your local grocery store or through a home delivery program or you had to read a book and follow their preset menus. N.F.J.—Not for Jennifer.

What the Weight Watchers *PointsPlus*® program does so well is it expands your options by teaching you to eat real food in the real world. It's so easy. You really can eat anything you want and it allows you necessary flexibility to keep you on the plan. And it teaches you how to implement activity that fits into your daily lifestyle without telling you that you absolutely have to hit the gym. It teaches behavior modification by helping you become aware of the bad food habits you've created that are holding you back. And finally, the program offers a tremendous amount of support through its meetings. For many, the meetings are where the rubber hits the road. They can make the difference between staying with the plan and leaving it.

While I wasn't able to attend as many traditional meetings as I would have liked to, when I did, I often found those to be truly inspirational. I was finally able to sit in a room with other people who were having the same struggles and challenges I was having. Hearing their stories was so helpful to know how other people were troubleshooting their problems and how they were receiving support from others. I found it so inspiring to meet other members who had been struggling with their weight for as long as I had been because it helped me come to a better understanding of my own journey. One member told me she had rejoined Weight Watchers fifteen times over the years. I couldn't believe it because I had become such an advocate for the program I could never imagine leaving! Still, she never gave up. She eventually came back and has finally found her stride. That is dedication.

Permanent weight loss doesn't come with an on and off switch. It is not something you do for a little while and think it is going to change your body. My schedule is as jam-packed as one can get and I still found the time to make the program work. You have to want weight-loss success so badly that no mountain, river, or ocean could keep you from reaching your goals. If you have that drive, passion, and commitment, there is no way you won't get there.

Whenever I couldn't make a traditional meeting, I always made time in my schedule to talk with Liz about my progress and my occasional frustrations. Amazingly, Liz was even able to meet me in South Africa for a few days when I was on location for four months shooting *Winnie*. There she introduced me to South African Weight Watchers leaders I could call on if I needed extra support. Liz was available when I needed her.

When I signed on to do the role of *Winnie*, I agreed to conform to the character, which meant losing weight before shooting and learning the proper dialect. I was already well on my way with the weight loss, so I wasn't concerned about meeting that requirement. I was, however, utterly terrified about learning the accent. I started working with a dialect coach two months before filming began. I wasn't familiar with the South African accent Winnie Mandela spoke with, but as an actress, I felt the burden of responsibility to get it right. I thought about Meryl Streep and all of the amazing characters she convincingly played throughout her career and used her as my inspiration to nail the language.

I never had the opportunity to meet Mrs. Mandela in person, but I knew she was an important figure in history and I wanted to honor her many worldly contributions. Playing her was not to be taken lightly, especially as an American actress portraying an African woman. I needed to be completely in the role, and for the first week or so, I was struggling with that. If I couldn't make that commitment, I wanted to do the right thing and pull myself from the film. Making *Winnie* was a huge and scary time in my life because of the immense nature of the character and because this was the first time I was separated from my baby for an extended period. My son was too young to make the trip to South Africa because going there requires a series of vaccinations. Also, David didn't want him to travel, which I completely understood. It was very far away, and not always terribly safe for such a young baby who is more vulnerable to infections and who cannot have the necessary inoculations. When I signed on for the project, I didn't have a family. But now I did. Being away from them was by far the hardest part of making the film.

When we started filming, I believe Darrell Roodt, the director of the movie, could tell I was struggling. He came to me one day to acknowledge that playing Winnie Mandela was a lot for anyone to take on. He said, "After everything you've been through and all that you've experienced—you're still here and that lets me know that you want to be here."

At the time, I couldn't see the forest for the trees, but I listened to Darrell and heard what he was trying to say. Whenever I'm in a situation, whether it is being eliminated from *American Idol* or up against 782 other actresses for a role, I have to fall back on my faith that God has a plan for me. God put me here, so I had no choice but to go with it. I will take that ride because I know it's my destiny. It took me another solid week to immerse myself in the role of Winnie, but once I did, I was in it to win it.

We shot the entire movie on location in South Africa, including Cape Town and Victoria. My days were long and deeply trying because the role was extremely emotional. I got up very early in the mornings, usually between four and five a.m., and didn't return back to my hotel until very late at night. If I had a day off, I used it to catch up on my sleep or take in the culture of the cities and tiny villages that surrounded me. Although the producers offered to take the cast on safari, I didn't want to do that. I was there to do a job, and when I wasn't working, I wanted to experience the local communities and meet the people. When I did, the conditions that I saw were beyond my understanding of poverty. On my way home from shooting one day, I looked out the car window and saw a little boy who was only slightly older than my baby, washing his underwear in a river. He seemed so happy and content. Despite his situation, I was struck by how joyful this boy appeared.

I saw townships where people lived in mud huts with thatched roofs, had no running water, no plumbing, no electricity, and no vegetation. I noticed smoke coming from one of the townships one day—that seemed odd. I thought there was a fire burning, but there wasn't. The smell of the smoke was so strong that it gave me a pounding headache. When I asked someone about it, they explained that this was the way those people warmed their homes. I was only exposed to the fumes for a short time and it made me sick; I couldn't imagine how the people who live in that township felt living with the smell every night. As we pulled away I saw two little girls out of the corner of my eye. They were both barefoot, walking on glass and dirt. I couldn't imagine letting my baby walk on the city streets of Chicago with no shoes, let alone the filth-laden roads these children were on. And still, those little girls just smiled and waved as we drove away. I asked someone from the crew if they could help me arrange to send shoes to all of the people in that area. And we did. When we returned to give them away, one woman fell to her knees crying because she finally had her own pair of shoes. In that moment, I suddenly realized how spoiled and shallow most people really are. Shortly before going to Africa, my makeup artist and I were in France for a fashion show and we were fussing over the fact that our hotel didn't have electrical outlets in the bathroom. After seeing how these people lived in Africa, I feel so foolish for acting that way. We live like royalty compared to the conditions I saw in Africa. In many ways, the experience there made me grow up. I learned so much about myself through the eyes of Winnie Mandela.

Aside from being away from my family, the hardest part of being in South Africa was trying to stay on the Weight Watchers program. This was the test of all tests on my weight-loss journey. Between the time change and the nature of my demanding production schedule, it was very hard to adjust to being there. The schedule hugely impacted my eating habits because my waking hours were much longer than when I am home, which meant I had to make my Points stretch throughout the day. This took some getting used to, especially because I was eating on the fly, and in between takes.

Thankfully, the portion sizes in this part of the world are much smaller than the enormous American sizes, their food production is less processed, and how food is delivered is so different. Instead of distributing overprocessed foods that can keep on a shelf longer, suppliers invested their money in better refrigeration and smarter packaging so they can package fresh foods. This worked to my advantage and was a real eye-opening experience for me. Because their emphasis was on offering fresher foods instead of foods laden with preservatives, I could continue to move away from the processed foods I had sometimes relied on before Weight Watchers and eat fresher, healthier foods. Even the food labels in South Africa were very different from the ones we have back in the United States, so I had to spend some time figuring out ingredients and calories. Because their country is on the metric system, the labels don't carry the same numbers I was used to, which meant I also had to learn to calculate my Points in a whole new way. But I did.

*Winnie* was challenging on so many levels. I was making a film that was filled with so much darkness and was deeply investing myself into my character. I was away from my family and found myself feeling sad, lonely, and depressed. As a result, I actually stopped eating enough food to maintain my weight. I was unintentionally losing more weight than I wanted to.

At the time I was actually as scared to lose more weight as I was to gain it. It was so outside of any scenario I had ever played out in my head. I didn't think there would ever be a day that Jennifer Hudson would be afraid of being too *skinny*. Thankfully, the Weight Watchers team was right there by my side helping me to figure things out so I didn't face a diet disaster. It took some convincing, but I actually had to start adding extra Points to my plan so I could maintain a healthy weight and look consistent on camera. I was eating more, but it was healthy food this time around.

I was so determined to get this—and not use being on location as an excuse to fall off my program. I understood the principles of Weight Watchers inside and out by now. There was no reason I couldn't take everything Weight Watchers had taught me and all of my experiences with me and make this work. If I could rise to the challenge, I could take my weight loss to the next level.

I really believe that it was my time and experience in South

Africa that solidified me as a person who actually lives a healthy lifestyle and no longer allows my environment to get in the way. And because of that, I finally *trusted the plan*. Completely. There is no doubt it works.

"*I got this*," I said aloud.

And I did.

As I grew more confident, I began to notice that people from the cast and crew were starting to pay attention to what I was doing. Several people began asking lots of questions about Weight Watchers and my personal program. The script supervisor used to bring me chocolate every single day on the set. She kept asking people how I could eat chocolate and still be so skinny. Someone finally told her that I track my food and then keep a tally of my Points. By doing this, I stay within my limits and won't fall away from the plan. Intrigued, she came to me to find out more about the Weight Watchers program. Before I knew it, I had several people from the movie following the plan, too. I suddenly felt like the Pied Piper leading the way.

After navigating my way through eating in South Africa, I now know that I can travel anywhere and stick to the program. It doesn't matter where you are because conscious eating is the same all over the world. Saying you can't because of where you are physically is just an excuse—covering up something going on emotionally or psychologically.

When I returned from South Africa, I was asked to shoot my

second commercial for Weight Watchers. I wanted to play a joke on the Weight Watchers people by wearing a fat suit in to the shoot so they would think I gained back all of my weight while I was on location. I couldn't get a convincing fat suit in time, so I did the next best thing. I wore a prosthetic pregnancy belly in to the shoot and had them all believing I was having another baby. Even my manager wasn't in on the joke, so when everyone saw me, they freaked, but no one said a word. I was sitting in a chair rubbing my tummy like I was ready to pop at any minute. When I got to wardrobe, the stylist took one look at me and said, "We may need to let your clothes out a bit. . . ." She was panicking because I was supposed to come in with a brand-new size-6 body. Instead, I came in looking nine months pregnant!

I couldn't believe that everyone was being so polite, especially because we only had that day to shoot the commercial.

Finally, the stylist looked at me and asked if I was pregnant.

"No. It's a joke." We had a good laugh over it, even if no one else did!

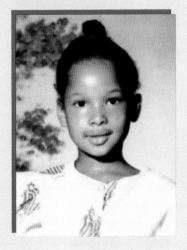

Me at age seven—I was always tall for my age.

The picture says it all!
Walter and me at prom.

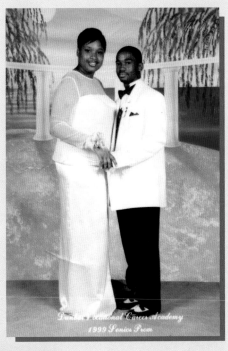

Prom night with Walter.
Big brother was definitely
watching.

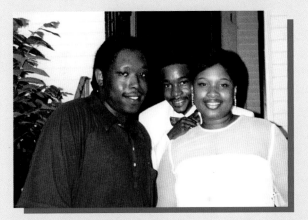

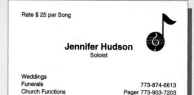

Rate $ 25 per Song

**Jennifer Hudson**
Soloist

Weddings
Funerals
Church Functions

773-874-6613
Pager 773-903-7203

$25 a song . . . now that was a bargain!

My dramatic velvet and silver gown from my talent show days.

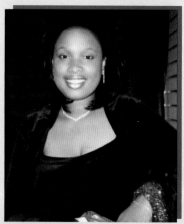

*Walter Williams III*

*Walter Williams III*

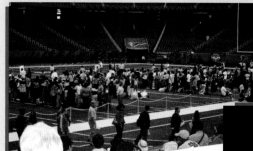

On the football field in Atlanta waiting for my first *American Idol* audition.

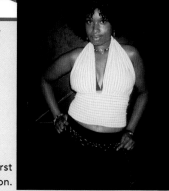

Ready to rock my first *American Idol* audition.

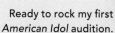

*Walter Williams III*

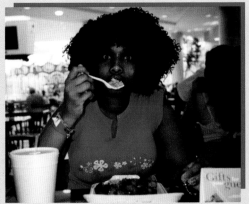

Feeding my face!

*Walter Williams III*

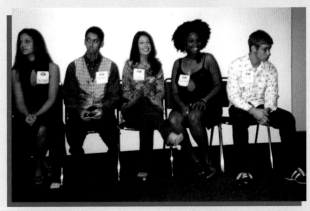

Waiting to audition for the judges—do you like my big hair?

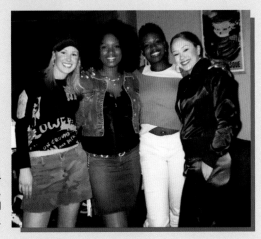

*American Idol* Season 3 top 24 contestants, Ashley Thomas, me, Fantasia Barrino, and Diana DeGarmo.

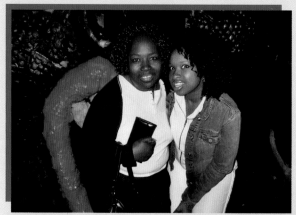

With Mama touring L.A.

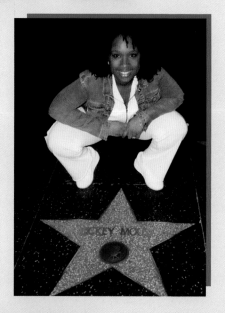

Dreaming of someday having
my own star—still waiting!

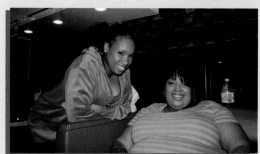

My sister Julia and me.

Celebrating my win for *Dreamgirls* at the Golden Globes.

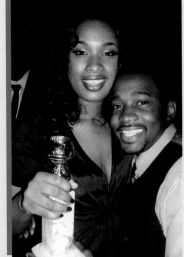

Walter Williams III

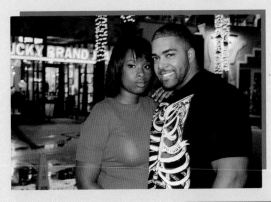

David and me in Boston.

Backstage at the Staples Center for Michael Jackson's memorial service with Usher, Stevie Wonder, and Magic Johnson.

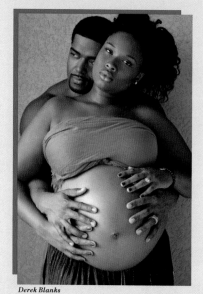

Derek Blanks

David and me shortly before the birth of our son.

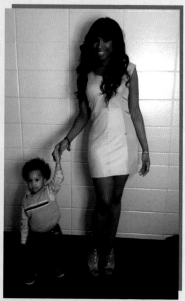

My baby and me.

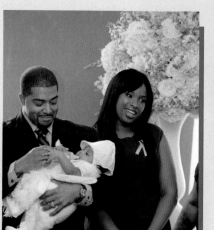

Derek Blanks

At David Jr.'s christening—a blessing for all of us.

Clive Davis and me.

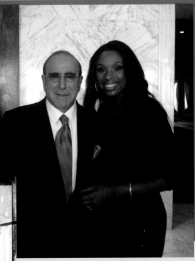

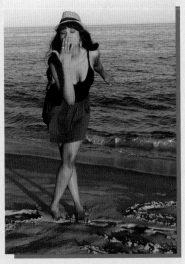

Something about this picture reminds me of Twiggy.

Walter and me now. We've come a long way together.

On the beach in the Hamptons, enjoying a rare day off.

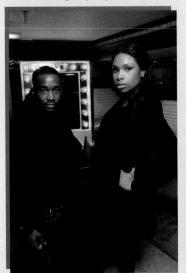

*Thomas Blue*

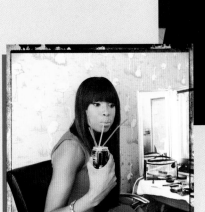

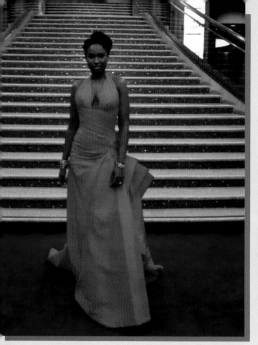

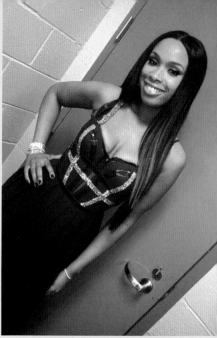

I loved my Versace gown that I wore to the 2011 Oscars.

Ready to rock the Grammys.

Getting ready for the Met Ball, wearing a Vera Wang gown.

I think I look hot!

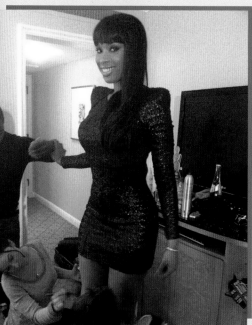

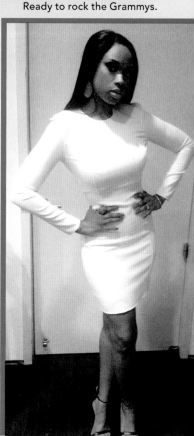

# CHAPTER TEN

# DON'T LOOK DOWN

Once I got into the groove, being on Weight Watchers actually became fun. I wanted to tell everyone I knew about how great I think this plan is for losing weight. Everywhere I go people stop and want to ask me how I lost my weight. Not long ago, I was in a park playing with my son when a young heavy-set girl came over to me.

"Wow. You look so skinny!" she said. "So, that Weight Watchers thing really works, huh?"

I was thrilled to take the time to talk to this young girl and tell her all about the virtues of the program. Even though I was at the park to spend time with my baby boy, if it meant that five minutes of my time could change a life, I was happy to share my journey with this perfect stranger.

"So, this is how it works. All you have to do is keep track of your Points. You get a certain number of Points to use each day. When you've used those up, you're done eating for the day. That's it. That's how I did it." I was trying to keep it as simple as I could.

"That sounds too hard," she said.

As soon as I heard her response, I knew this girl wasn't ready to make the commitment to change. One thing I know for sure is, you can't force the issue. When someone wants to lose weight, they will do whatever it takes. They can't do it for anyone else but themselves. It has to be for them alone. Without that understanding, they will fail.

As my weight loss progressed, I shared my newfound love for healthy eating with my sister and several other members of my family. My family has always been supportive of everything I do, so when I told everyone that I had started Weight Watchers, several of them decided that they wanted to try it, too. And for those who wouldn't get on board, Lord knows, I did what I could to try to convince them to join.

## JULIA, MY SISTER

Our family is a family that eats. If you go to anyone's house for a visit, they will always try to feed you. That's the way it has always been. When my sister, Jenny, decided to go on Weight Watchers, she came to me and begged me to start the program with her. Jenny was always the skinny-mini in our family. Maybe it's because Jason and I were so much heavier than her that we never noticed that Jenny was heavy, too. She told me all about Liz, her weight-loss leader, and offered to set up a consultation between us. I wasn't all that into going, but I told my cousin Pam about my meeting, hoping she might want to come with me. Before I knew it, several other family members decided to join us, too. I was still reluctant, but since the family was getting on board, I agreed to give the program a try. I was very successful for the first two months. Before I knew it, I was down forty pounds, and after years of insulin dependence, I noticed that when I was eating according to the Weight Watchers plan, I really didn't have to take my daily shots. You might think that that was enough to keep me motivated to stick with it, but it wasn't. Aside from the change in my blood sugar levels, I didn't really feel any different from the weight loss, plus my old eating habits were really hard to break.

I know that no one was holding me back but me, and still, I couldn't seem to follow through. You see, I am an expert excuse-maker, so I came up with a thousand reasons I didn't want to stay with the plan. I drive a bus, which means I sit on my rear end all day long. Most everyone I know who drives a bus for a living gains weight. Since I have to get up really early in the morning to make my shift, I don't have enough time to prepare my food for the day. I'd stop at the gas station on my way in and buy chips and donuts to eat for breakfast. Truth be told, I enjoy eating junk food. I've always been that way and don't have any plans to give it up. The funny thing is, I am the most competitive person in our family. If I really gave my all, I know I'd be the family's biggest loser. My head is just not there. I don't like it when someone tells me I can't do something, so restricting how much of my favorite foods I could eat just didn't work for me.

I think about going back to meetings. I see the progress that Jenny and so many of my other relatives have made, so deep down, I know the plan works. If I ever go back, I will have to commit to getting it together, and right now, I don't really have the willpower to do that—at least not yet. One thing is for sure, if our mama were here, she'd be fussing over Jenny's weight loss. She'd say something like, "Now, Jenny, you just got too skinny and don't be losing any more weight!" That would be our mama.

My sister and I have always been close but we couldn't be more opposite—especially when it comes to taking care of our bodies and our health. She loves her junk food, and though I love my food, too, these days I like it healthy. I've always been known for my strong beliefs, but my sister has that dangerous combination of being both strong and stubborn. I tell her all the time that she needs to try a new way of looking at food and change her eating habits or she will not be around to enjoy life. She's so feisty when she is telling me she is "fine," and that she doesn't need my advice. But the reality is, she is very overweight and suffers from diabetes. She is completely insulin dependent, in part due to her obesity. I love my sister and want her to be around for a long time. I had hoped that she would somehow get inspired by my weight loss and give Weight Watchers a try for herself. I begged and begged until one day she finally said she would do it. Julia stayed on the program for two months and lost a little more than forty pounds. But then she quit.

I was so proud of her effort and disappointed in her decision to stop. If she really gave it her all, Julia could blow my results right out of the water because her weight loss would be far more dramatic. She knows she's the only one holding herself back, and when she gets sick and tired of feeling the way she does, she will come back. I know it.

I think Julia is like a lot of women who want to lose weight. They give it their all for a while, but they don't fully change their habits. Anyone can lose a few pounds, but not everyone has the tools to stick with it. I don't judge my sister for giving up. I understand her feelings, and I feel her pain and frustration. I know how hard it is to undo everything you know and are comfortable with doing—especially when you have a lot of weight to lose. It feels like a huge mountain you have to climb. But we can't let our insecurities own or destroy us. We have to face them head-on. That was part of the challenge that motivated me to take this journey. I wanted to see what I could do and, more important, I wanted to understand everything that was holding me back. That took some soul-searching and spending some time alone asking myself the hard questions we all avoid.

"What makes me feel this way?"

"Why do I choose to make poor food choices?"

"What is my core problem?"

Until you can answer those types of questions, you will keep making excuses that only you view as your roadblocks to success. We all make up excuses as a way of avoiding something we don't want to do. Excuses are our way of making a decision okay for ourselves.

How do I know this?

Because I was once there.

I was that person.

I had that mind-set, so I am well aware of why that type of thinking only holds us back.

When my very first Weight Watchers commercial came out, people freaked out because I was sitting in a chair wearing a blazer.

"She didn't lose weight."

"She's sitting down. Who can tell what she looks like?"

These were the types of comments people made about me. But in reality, these were just excuses they were making for themselves. They are the same excuses Julia is still making and the ones I made for myself over the years. That is why I can identify it for what it was.

When the second commercial came along, my stylist kept me in that damn jacket, so people still doubted my progress. It reminded me of getting the role of Effie in *Dreamgirls*. I heard so many people say, "She got the part, but I bet she can't sing the music," and, "She can sing, but can she act?"

People! Stop!

For all of those doubters, haters, and excuse-makers out there— listen up because I've got something to say.

Hear this loud and clear.

*I am completely in charge of the choices I make about what I am doing to lose weight and get healthy.*

And you know what? We *all* have this power.

Don't be angry with me for something good I've done for myself. Be angry with yourself for not having the courage to do the same in your own life.

At the end of the day, you're not hurting me—you're hurting yourself.

So, stop pointing the finger at everyone else.

Stop making excuses about why you "can't."

And start taking action.

The same frame of mind that is keeping you from doing it is the mind that will help you to achieve what you want to do.

If you're at home reading this book and asking yourself why I have this success and you don't, don't be angry with me—stop and ask yourself what your issues are that are holding you back. Don't be afraid of the answers. Be afraid of not asking the questions.

My cousin Gina started Weight Watchers the same time I did. Every time I saw her, I was losing weight and she wasn't. She'd make comments like, "You're skinny and I can't stand you," while complaining that the program wasn't working for her.

"Girl, you know you're not working the program. If you were, you'd be skinny, too!" Then I told her to stop her complaining and get into the right mind-set so she could do it. When she finally made up her mind to lose the weight, it fell off just like that. If you can break down those walls you've spent so many years building to protect yourself, you can achieve anything.

Are you still making excuses or are you ready to make a change?

And speaking of change, I never thought I'd see the day that my entire family would gravitate toward something like losing weight. It still blows my mind. I often ask myself, Is this the same family? Everyone from the women and the men, the young and the old, is finally consciously aware of what they are putting in their bodies and want to make the right choices. Remember, I come from a family where food was a major part of every gathering and where the women would get on your case if they thought you were getting too thin. A family that loved a table full of fried chicken, pork chops, biscuits, and gravy.

Our biggest success story so far is my cousin Pam, whom we lovingly refer to as our "biggest loser" because she has lost more than one hundred and five pounds so far (and counting). It had been a while since I had seen Pam, so after she lost around seventy-five pounds, I invited her to come see me at one of my shows. I saw this girl trailing me backstage but didn't realize it was *my cousin*. I was only able to recognize her by the sound of her voice. I told her how amazing I thought she looked—and she did.

## PAM CURB, MY COUSIN

Like a lot of women, I had slowly put on weight throughout the years without totally noticing just how much I'd gained. One morning I stepped on the scale, and much to my surprise, it read 337 pounds! "No way!" I said out loud. The scale had to be wrong. I was expecting to see somewhere around three hundred pounds, but not 337.

Now you might think that weighing three hundred an extra thirty-seven pounds wouldn't much matter, but it did. Every time I went to the doctor over the years, I always let them weigh me, but I never allowed them to tell me the number on the scale. I'd avoided it for so long that I lost track of my weight.

I didn't think it was possible that I had gained more than one hundred pounds since my wedding day thirteen years back. I didn't realize that I was that big. I got a little weepy-eyed because I had let myself go that far without paying any attention to how I looked or felt.

The truth is, I was tired all of the time. I chalked that up to getting up early for work, taking care of my three children, and running around all the time. I didn't have the energy to do any of it with gusto. When my three-year-old wanted me to play with her, I couldn't. She became intentionally defiant when I was scolding her. I'd say, "Come here right now," but she wouldn't move because she knew there was no way I was going to chase her. I couldn't.

We were all at a family gathering when Jen walked through the door looking like a model. "Girl, what are you doing? Tell me now!" She said she had gone on

Weight Watchers. I had been on their plan before and didn't believe her because I hadn't lost a pound when I tried. But Jenny kept telling me how easy the program was, and by looking at her, it obviously works.

A few months later, I saw Jenny again. This time she had lost even more weight. I was mesmerized by how she looked.

"Pam, if someone gave you a book and told you to stay within these Points and you will lose weight while still eating anything you want, would you tell them no?" Jenny asked.

"I guess not," I said.

That same night, the Lord spoke to me. "You aren't going to be here for your kids."

When I told my husband, Mario, about the message I had received, he said, "We want you to be here, Pam, and if you don't make some changes, you won't be." He was right.

Shortly after that, Liz came to meet with some of our family members to get us all started. I was eager to jump on the bandwagon and give it a try. Liz explained the program to me in great detail. I immediately thought there was no way I could ever do it because I didn't have time to count my Points. The reality is that I wasn't sure I was ready to give the plan a chance. Liz assured me that I was feeling like many of her members—overwhelmed. And she was right. "Then just change one thing, Pam. Weight Watchers is a lifetime journey. Tell me one thing you are going to change for this week and I promise that you will see results." I had to think about it for a second. When I told Liz that I ate chips for breakfast, she said, "That's not breakfast food." And she was right. For the next week, I made a conscious decision to eat better. I told my husband, Mario, that I was going to give Weight Watchers a try and if he wanted to help me lose weight, then he had to help me with the plan. So he woke up at 3:00 in the morning to fix me a bag of food to take to work. He boiled eggs for me, gave me apples, carrots, and all sorts of healthy choices to pick from. I wasn't used to preparing my breakfast or lunch, so Mario's help meant the world to me.

Mario had noticed I had gained the weight over the years but he never said a word. He wanted me to lose the weight but never really pushed me. He encouraged me to get healthy, which I didn't understand meant losing weight. He inspired me every day by reminding me that I didn't have to be full, only satisfied. He helped me curb my desire to go back for second helpings, something I never thought twice about before starting Weight Watchers. These days I have to make sure that I measure out my portions or I will still overeat.

I told my mother, husband, and children that I wanted to take a year and focus on taking care of myself so I could finally get healthy. They were all on board with that decision and said they would do whatever they could to help me get there. My husband got me started on taking walks around the neighborhood. He was committed to helping me on my journey any way he could. I was the luckiest wife on the planet because some husbands aren't as supportive or involved. My mother helped out by making healthy dinners for us after I put in long days at work and didn't have the time to cook for us myself. If I didn't have everyone's help, I am not sure I could have stayed with the program all on my own. My success has come from the love and encouragement I've received from all of my family.

Once I started exercising, I realized that I had to make the time to do that every day. It didn't matter where or when as long as I got ten minutes of movement in. Since I drive a bus, I knew I had time while waiting in the lineup. I started running up and down the aisle of the bus until the passengers started loading. Sometimes I'd park the bus while waiting and walk around it for those ten minutes. My passengers began to notice what I was doing and were encouraging me to keep up the good work. The more I worked out, the better I felt, and my results were even more significant. I eventually joined a health club to take my fitness to the next level. My husband joined, too, so I would have a workout partner to keep me motivated.

Weight Watchers is the easiest plan I have ever been on. I didn't have to deny myself anything. If I wanted to eat a piece of cake without feeling bad, I could as long as I calculated in the Points for my day. Over the course of a year or so, I lost seventy-five pounds and felt great. My knees were no longer an issue; I had more energy and could breathe a lot easier. It was right around that weight that I hit a plateau in my loss. I began getting careless with tracking my Points. I was messing up every day and couldn't seem to get back on track. Liz reminded me that every day was a new chance to start over, so once I could get my head back into the game, I was able to focus and get back to the plan. As Liz so often reminded me, eating healthy is a lifetime journey. People think of Weight Watchers as a diet, but it isn't. It is a way of eating you want to commit to for life. Not long ago, one of my co-workers saw me eating lunch and asked, "Are you still eating healthy?"

My answer was simple: "I have made a commitment to myself to turn my life around and this is part of it."

To date, I've lost one hundred and five pounds. I've got fifty more to go. I don't have a set weight goal, but I want to get down to a size 12 or 14. When I get there, I'll be happy. My husband is grateful, too, because as he says, "I've got my wife back."

My aunt Bae Mae is in her seventies and has lost more than forty-six pounds. I had only ever known Aunt Bae Mae as a big woman. She was so inspired by my weight loss that she decided to give it a try, too. I think she's the true inspiration for making a decision to take control of her health and weight so late in life. If she can make that decision at her age, there is simply no excuse for anyone else to say they can't do it. I was especially stunned when I heard that my uncle Charles, who is known as the barbecue man in our family because his brother once owned his own barbecue restaurant, is sitting in weekly Weight Watchers meetings, losing weight, too. These two relatives are living proof that it is never too late to get control of your health.

## AUNT BAE "BABY" MAE

### Age 74

I began my journey with Weight Watchers in May 2010 after one of my cousins called me to say she had started on their program. At the time, I wasn't thinking about losing weight. I've never been a big eater, but I like rich food. I rather enjoy eating grits, greens with salt pork or ham hock, but most of all, I really like butter. And as they say, "Everything is better with butter!" Still, I'd been a big woman my entire life and at my age, I thought, What's the point? She tried to entice me by telling me that the Weight Watchers people were coming to talk to everyone in the family and we were going to have our picture taken to track our progress. "Picture? I don't want any pictures taken!" I told her the only way I would join her was if she took a bus trip with me to an upcoming family reunion. She said, "If I go with you, will you try the program with me?" I reluctantly said I would try it for a week or two.

So many members of our family had started on the Weight Watchers plan that they held their own meetings every week at our church. I really enjoyed attending those meetings because they inspired me. When I heard other people's stories and saw how well my family members were doing on the plan, I felt like I could do it, too.

I lost two or three pounds the first week on the plan. That was enough to get me to go back to another meeting and see how I could do better during week two. I gave up drinking excessive amounts of cola like I used to and replaced it with water. I was amazed that I could eat all types of food as long as I ate them in the right portions. It took me some time to realize that I could no longer go back for a second hamburger, but at least I could still eat one if I wanted to. Today I still eat my beloved grits, but now I'll have a half of a cup instead of a heaping spoonful serving—I get the flavor without all of the unwanted extra Points. I won't bring my old favorite foods into the house, and though my husband still drinks his soda pop, I keep it in the basement where it is out of sight, out of mind, so I won't be tempted. And even if I were, as a senior person, I am not walking those stairs unless I have to!

I'm a Christian woman, who believes that the Lord always has a plan. When I joined Weight Watchers I realized that, like my faith, the door is open for all those who will come. You have to accept the plan and realize that if you slip, and you might, you can't use that as a reason to give up or stop. Even if you go a week without losing a pound, be happy that you didn't gain one. Eating healthy is a continuous way of life. We're all human, which means we will make mistakes. Don't dwell on that—focus on getting back to eating right and you will feel so good.

Even my twelve-year-old cousin Star has benefited from the program. Her story is very near and dear to me because she is a young girl with a bundle of talent who has always been a little chubby and didn't have the self-esteem to see herself as the beautiful girl she truly is. Her mother came to me a while back to ask my thoughts on how to break her daughter into the music business. I knew from my own experiences that there is so much competition out there, and like it or not, my cousin was going to be judged on her appearance before her talent. Lord knows I had lived through that scene too many times in my life. I encouraged her mother, who was also a Weight Watchers member, to share with Star the new healthy habits from the program. That way Star could face the competition that she was up against with a fair shot of breaking out. Star said she was scared to make changes. Discouraged by Star's refusal, her mom asked me to talk to her, hoping that I might be able to convince her to listen to the advice and learn how to eat healthy.

I spoke with Star for about an hour. I reminded her of all of her positive assets. I told her that no one is perfect—no one. We always think the grass is greener on the other side, but the reality is that everyone struggles with something. I laughed as I shared my thoughts on how everyone has a shape. Some girls have great shapes while others are built like boys. Both are still shapes. Some are built like two-liter bottles of soda and others are built like single cans.

"You know what? I was once that bottle!" I said. I think she knew what I meant.

As we talked, I assured her that no one needed to know she was changing her eating habits and that she could go at her own pace. Before we went our separate ways, I committed to becoming her mentor throughout her journey and promised that she wouldn't go through any of these changes alone.

I didn't have anyone to guide me like that when I was her age, but I was determined to break that cycle in our family by making myself available to anyone who had the desire to get healthy. I managed to talk her into listening to what her mother had to say, and guess what? It worked! She is a whole new person; she can see herself for the amazing girl she is. While her outer appearance has definitely changed, it is her inner beauty that is finally shining through.

Altogether, seventy-five of my family members have gone on the program and, as of the writing of this book, they have collectively lost more than *two thousand* pounds. They attend a weekly

Weight Watchers meeting where they all get together to support one another through their journeys. One of the most valuable lessons I learned from Liz was the importance of having a solid support system. That lack of support is one of the biggest reasons people gain back the weight they have worked so hard to take off. Weight Watchers was so impressed by my family members and their commitment to the program that they actually put two of my cousins in a television commercial for the company in an effort to make their weight loss real for everyday people. Ultimately, weight loss and getting healthy have become a real family affair.

It blows me away to see these people taking control of their health because our family has always loved food—especially unhealthy food. It's such a change in lifestyle for everyone, especially the elders in my family, who never dieted a day in their lives. When I threw my son's second birthday party, almost everyone attending asked me to plan a special Weight Watchers–friendly menu so they could stay on the plan that day. As I walked around the party, we all began talking about our personal weight-loss journeys, and we created a spontaneous Weight Watchers meeting on the spot.

"Jenny, how many Points are in this burger?"

"Can I eat this?"

"Help me not fall off today . . ."

I suddenly felt like I was a Weight Watchers leader, and I loved every minute of the joyful experience. Seeing so many of my relatives enthusiastically embrace these changes makes me feel like Jesus has a bigger plan for me outside of music.

Sharing this moment was amazing. I felt more proud that day than I did receiving my Oscar. For real. Part of my drive to keep at it myself is so I can continue to set a positive example for my family and others.

Healthy eating is a choice, a lifestyle, and a decision only you can make for yourself, but once you do, you'll never want to go back to the way you used to feel.

Even though I have been extremely public about my commitment to Weight Watchers, some people still think I lost the weight by some other means. Some even believe that I had gastric bypass surgery. Here's the thing. I am all about doing things in a natural way. My sister came to me a while ago to say she wanted to have her stomach stapled. I was all over her before she finished the sentence.

"Julia. That's cheating. It's the lazy way out and I won't let you do that. You have to want to lose the weight and then do the work for it to truly mean anything." And that is how I really feel. So when people ask me how I took off my excess pounds, I tell them I did it the old-fashioned way—with determination and commitment. And just so we're completely clear about what I am saying, whenever you see my stretch marks and excess skin—that is to let you know that my weight loss is real. I am proud of those reminders of how I once looked. They are my war wounds, my battle scars, and they're there to remind me of what used to be the truth. A truth I created and a truth I changed. If I had any type of cosmetic surgery, don't you think I'd get that stuff fixed, too? Of course I would! But I didn't. I didn't do anything but eat right and exercise. You can take that to the bank. And you can do it, too.

*According to a recent OECD study, in the United States, the cost of treating obesity-related diseases, such as diabetes, heart disease, and stroke, will increase $66 billion per year by 2030, and represent a 2.6 percent increase in overall health spending. The increasing rates of obesity would mean 7.8 million extra cases of diabetes, 6.8 million extra cases of coronary heart disease and stroke, and 539,000 extra cancer cases by 2030. Losing just a little weight could offset those increases. The report noted that a 1 percent population-wide decrease in body-mass index (just 1.9 pounds for an average 198-pound adult) would prevent more than 2 million cases of diabetes, roughly 1.5 million cases of heart disease and stroke, and 73,000 to 127,000 cancer cases in the United States.*

Not only did Weight Watchers change the way I thought about food; it altered my entire way of thinking. I became a much more organized person because I had to practice structure about my meals and keep meticulous notes on what I ate every single day. And even though many experts will tell you not to weigh yourself daily, it's now the first thing I do every morning. I weigh completely naked so there is nothing that can mysteriously add an unexpected pound here or there other than my food intake. This routine helps me to control my fluctuations in weight. If I see a small gain, I know I can do something about it that day. I can drink more water and make smarter food choices to move the needle on that scale back down. I try to weigh myself only in the morning because doing so at other times of the day can have slight fluctuations. Doing this helps keep the circumstances the same each time, so I feel as if I am getting an accurate weight. I know I'm not alone in this—it is just a human compulsion.

If I don't get on the scale every day, I feel as if I am not on top of my progress or lack thereof. If I check into a hotel and my room doesn't have a scale, I call housekeeping to bring one up. Call it a habit or an obsession—either way, I have to know where I am on the scale at all times. If I've gained a pound or two and don't know it, there is nothing preventing me from continuing to gain weight, especially if I am unaware of that movement in the first place. I also do my weekly Weight Watchers weigh-ins like all members, just not usually at meetings. Everyone has their own method of gauging where they're at. Some people never get on the scale and merely go by how their clothes are fitting, while others obsess over the number they see at their feet every day. I am one of those obsessed people. Hello. My name is Jennifer and yes, I am addicted to the scale.

By late 2009, I was back in the studio recording my second album, *I Remember Me*. The title track is based on a poem I wrote one morning because I wanted to share how I felt about all of the experiences I have had, including the highs and the lows and everything in between. The song was written to allow people to get to know and then embrace the new me. I had been through so much throughout my career, in my personal life, and during my weight loss that I wanted to reconnect with my fans by giving them some insight about how all of that felt. I felt like a new person, but I was still the same girl.

While recording the album, I got to work with the incredibly talented R. Kelly, who wrote my first single, "Where You At." R. Kelly really got me. Although we both live in Chicago, we had never met while making the album. Even so, he somehow understood me.

I also got to work with the fantastic Alicia Keys, who wrote "Angel" and cowrote "Don't Look Down" and "Everybody Needs Love"; and one of my favorite songwriters, Diane Warren, whom I had previously worked with on "Still Here" for my first album, but made it onto my second album instead. "Still Here" was originally dedicated to my grandmother, but it really relates to my whole family. It's a way to remember and keep them in my life.

Diane's songs are the type of music I love to sing. When it comes to songwriting, she is in a league of her own. We recently collaborated on a song for the sound track of *Winnie* called "Bleed for Love." It is such a beautiful song. Give me a Diane Warren song any day of the week and I will smother it with Jennifer Hudson singing love.

I had purposely kept a pretty low profile while recording my second album. The first time I publicly revealed my partial weight loss was when I was asked to participate in a tribute to Whitney Houston at the 2010 BET Honors, held in Washington, D.C. As you can imagine, that was a treat for me. I was finally able to show my appreciation for Whitney by singing one of her biggest hits and most difficult songs to perform—"I Will Always Love You." That song meant so much to me that I told producers they had to let me do that song or I wouldn't perform at all! At the time, I had lost about thirty or so pounds. Although it wasn't that much, the change in my appearance was drastic. I wore a custom-made dress that hugged my body and showed off my brand-new shape.

When I came out onstage, I received a standing ovation based on my look alone. I hadn't even begun to sing. I had to look behind me to see if someone else had come out on the stage, too, because I couldn't understand why they were on their feet. I didn't realize it was just me they were screaming for. I think everyone was shocked by the change in my appearance. It felt unreal.

Ironically, before that night, there had actually been rumors circulating that I might be pregnant again. Those were quickly put to rest the moment I stepped out on the stage. It was one of the first moments I realized the tables had turned—audiences were still looking at me before listening to me, but for the first time in my career, my image was competing with my talent in a positive way.

I killed the song and gave Whitney every ounce of my blood, sweat, and tears that night. When I finished, the crowd went crazy, standing and cheering for me again for several minutes afterward. It was a wonderful feeling because this time, they were clapping for my art.

# CHAPTER ELEVEN

# I REMEMBER ME

I didn't realize how special growing up in Chicago was until I stepped out and lived someplace else for a while. At the end of the day, Chicago is my home. In many ways, it represents who I am, where I come from, and where I got started, and it gives me a sense of comfort I don't get anywhere else on the planet. When I'm in Chicago, I can just relax and be my old self, Jenny Kate. I can shop, walk the streets, and be myself without anyone making an unnecessary fuss. I know the good people of Chicago and they know me. And that familiarity helps me to feel safe, secure, and stay grounded in an otherwise crazy world that isn't known for those values.

Since David and I come from Chicago, both of our families are there, and family is something that is extremely important to both of us. That is why we made the decision to pack up our baby son and our three dogs, Oscar, Grammy, and Dream, and move our family back to our hometown in October 2010. I want him to have the same sense of family, tradition, and support that I grew up with. It was definitely time to go home.

Although Liz and Weight Watchers had somewhat prepared me for the physical changes I could expect to see in my body and then how to maintain those changes, no one really told me about the emotional acceptance, or even rejection, of losing weight and all of the emotional changes that would take place. She said that some people have such a hard time adjusting to their weight loss that they actually prefer to go back to the way they used to be by gaining back the pounds they lost and, for many, packing on even more. I am lucky that I have a good support system to help me deal with these feelings.

I knew there would be challenges along the way, but I welcome the opportunity to learn and grow from the experiences. "Bring it on!" That is always my attitude.

*In the United States, about one-quarter of all men were obese in 2008 regardless of their race, while 46 percent of black women, one-third of Hispanic women, and 30 percent of white women were obese.*

First, let me say that I love the way I look. I always have. But I am extremely proud of the hard work I've put into my weight loss and the effort I've given to getting healthy for my family. Nothing prepared me for the attention I now get as a result of losing weight. Even people I'm close to have had a hard time accepting my new shape, including my fiancé. If David had his way, he'd keep me dressed in flowing mumus all the time. To be honest, he doesn't really like it when I wear something that shows off my body. If I try to put on a pair of shorts that he thinks are too short, he freaks out. I think it's kind of funny because my man makes his living wearing drawers and nothing else. Why is it okay for him and not for me?

David has always been the type of man who tells me what he thinks, that I am beautiful, and that he loves when I don't wear makeup. He likes me best when I am plain.

Every now and then David will make comments that "his old girlfriend" never dressed in tight clothes or wore a lot of makeup. Of course, he is referring to me before I lost the weight. Sometimes, when we go out to eat, he'll occasionally offer me bites of whatever he's having, knowing I don't want to add the extra Points into my day. Sometimes I think he'd love to stuff me back to my old weight because it was what he was used to.

In all fairness, even I had to get into a new mind-set when it came to my body. I'd go shopping and reach for the same old sizes I've always grabbed for. Walter usually stopped me by saying, "That won't fit you—you're not a size twelve anymore." And he was right. Like I've said, I always had a shape, but this was the first time in my life that I had a skinny waist and a bra size that was smaller than I'd been since I first grew breasts!

Ever since *Dreamgirls*, designers have graciously sent me dresses to wear on the red carpet, but it was tricky because it was much harder then to find something to wear that fit, let alone flattered my body. The designers that made dresses in the larger sizes wanted to clothe me because they hardly ever got the chance to fit a "big girl." You can bet that Gwyneth Paltrow or Angelina Jolie and I were never fighting over the same dress.

These days, it's hard to pick out which dress I'm going to wear because they all look and fit amazingly. Still, I find it a little intimidating at times because I am not used to someone like Vera Wang asking me to wear one of her dresses at an event, Donatella Versace dressing me for the Oscars, or Michael Kors calling me up to see if I would like to wear one of his gowns at a private dinner in Rome. All I had to do was fly to Italy, put on his gown, have dinner, and mingle among the guests. Mary J. Blige was going to be there performing, too. Talk about coming from the whole other side of the rainbow.

I was someone who grew up never being looked at as a fashionista. And now, for the first time ever, I was actually going to be a model talking about what I was wearing! While you know I always saw myself as a supermodel, I must admit that I worried I might be a complete disaster if the dress didn't go over well. If I agreed to do it, I was purposefully and willingly putting myself in a place where I only was being judged on my physical appearance and nothing else. While I certainly had my share of dealing with that, it was never an intentional decision. It was a lot of pressure to consider. I thought, What the hell? I told Michael it would be an honor to wear his gown and had the best time ever doing it.

People I knew before I lost weight started looking at me in a whole new way. My friend and stylist Eric Archibald kept trying to dress me in the same type of clothes as he did before I lost the weight. He wanted to cover me up by putting me in a suit jacket. I felt like I was back on *American Idol.*

"I could have worn that jacket eighty pounds ago!" I loudly protested. "From now on, I only want to wear clothes that have a shape to them. That decision is final!" It is a good thing that Eric and I get each other and I know his heart is always in the right place, even if his clothing choice isn't!

Eric had been a fan of mine since I did *Dreamgirls.* He has the most amazing fashion sense of any stylist I have ever worked with. He gets what I like and what I don't like and how I feel about my body. Still, it took him a little while to come around to my new shape because he had grown so protective over my former body size. He used to refuse to put me in tight, formfitting clothes because he was concerned that I would be too self-conscious wearing them. What I discovered was, when I was heavier, he had his own insecurities about my size that he was inadvertently imposing on me. Honestly, I never felt self-conscious about my body. Never. My decision to lose weight was about being healthy for my son, not about changing my appearance to fit into some preconceived idea of what I should look like. I'd get so mad when Eric refused to bring me figure-flattering dresses because it was his way of telling me he didn't think I could wear that style. And y'all know I don't like it when someone tells me I can't do something. There's nothing that will make me put that dress on faster than someone telling me I shouldn't.

When I was picking a dress to wear to a 2011 pre-Oscar party, it seemed everyone had an opinion on whether I should wear the one I chose or not. Granted, it was short—even for me—but I didn't think it was *too* short.

"You can't wear that!" Walter said as he shook his index finger at me in total disapproval.

"Why not?" I knew what he was thinking, but every now and then I like to play with Walter to see him squirm.

"It's too . . . short!"

We bantered back and forth for a few minutes before I made

him take a picture with my iPhone so we could send it to my sister for her opinion. If Julia said it was too short, I'd agree to change into another dress. If she said it was fine, I had my outfit for the party.

"It looks great," she texted back, and with her approval I proudly wore that sizzling dress.

What was fascinating about this was that Walter is with me most every day. Even though he was a part of my weight-loss journey, like Eric, he also hadn't adjusted how he sees me. My sister has mostly seen the changes in my body from afar. Every time she saw a photo of me in a magazine or on the Internet, she saw drastic differences in my shape. I think the distance gave her a fresh perspective that the people closest to me on a daily basis simply didn't have—yet. They'd eventually come around, but oh, it wasn't easy. Walter is still trying to dress me like his grandma!

E ven though I have lost a lot of weight, I am still the same girl who felt self-conscious having to kiss Jamie Foxx in my first scene in *Dreamgirls*. I am still the same Jennifer I always was. I don't want to go and put everything out there on display just because I'm proud of the work I've done to lose weight. When I shot my music video for "No One's Gonna Love You" from my second album, I worked with a director who wanted to put me in super-sexy skin-baring outfits. She thought I would want to be exposed and show off my body. Now, I had never met this woman prior to the shoot, so she didn't know anything about me before making this decision.

Big mistake.

Big.

No one is going to make a decision about what I wear without running it by me first.

When it came time to do the first shot, she walked over to me and said, "Jennifer—for this video, you are so in love with your man that you just want to sleep with him."

*Say what?*

So here's how this goes. I hadn't been very involved with the planning of this particular video, so I didn't really know what the full story line was until I got to the set. My record company had hired the production team and created a storyboard with the director without my input. There had never been an instance in my career where I worried that someone would want to put me in a compromising position that didn't mesh with my image or brand—until *that* day.

The notion of me playing a sex kitten was a real eye-opener. Was my record label actually trying to repackage me and change how people saw me now that I had lost weight?

I had never done anything like that before my weight loss and I wasn't about to do it now, either. I changed every scene as we went along. I told them I would not cooperate with anything that didn't feel right to me. I made that pretty tough for everyone, all in the name of not compromising who I am. I'm not sorry. I am an adult, a mother, and a woman in charge of herself.

I am in control of all decisions that have to do with my image, which means that no one will decide what's right for me except me. I'm not special. We should all feel this way about ourselves. Sadly, so many women don't, and in the process they compromise their value to please someone else.

Sure, some people want to step out there and expose themselves by using their bodies to get ahead. That's not who I am. I know my value and wasn't about to taint my image for a record. I didn't need a sexy body to land the role of Effie, I didn't need a sexy body to win an Oscar, I didn't need a sexy body to win a Grammy, and I surely don't need a sexy body to make a music video.

I may have a new body but I am still the same person.

There are a whole lot of people out there who have applauded me for taking control of my weight and health. I've met so many women who have come up to say how much I have inspired them to take control of their health, too. They see my decision as strong and fearless because I stepped out of my comfort zone to reinvent myself. To those women, I want to say thank you. But I didn't really reinvent who I am so much as how I appear.

When I step out onto the stage, I can see and hear people react.

"Oh, my God—she looks amazing!"

"I had no idea she lost so much weight!"

"She is fabulous. I am so happy for her." And so on.

I actually open my shows with me behind a curtain in silhouette so the crowd can see me, get their comments in and done, and then I can do what they came there to see—entertain. For the most part, once they've checked me out, it's all good and the show goes on as usual.

But there has been another reaction people have had to my weight loss that came as quite a surprise to me. They say some very negative things. I'm serious. They are rejecting me instead of embracing me for getting healthy. Even the media began writing articles that I had taken my weight loss too far by losing way too much weight. One article accused me of "pulling a disappearing act," saying that I was "so svelte in my tangerine orange Versace dress at the 2011 Oscars, I nearly vanished when I turned to the side." Well, at least they didn't say it was too tight!

Apparently, there is a fine line in the media between being thin enough to succeed and being so thin that nutritionists I've never met actually worry about my health in the press. While I wasn't seeking publicity for my weight loss, it appears there are those who find it necessary to comment about me. Just as I had to go through a transition period, I guess they did, too. The funny thing is, I know my people, the fans who come see my shows, and up until I lost my weight, the audience was always filled with love and support. Now I've got people looking at me up onstage thinking they don't know me anymore. They see a thinner version of the girl they once knew and appreciated and are now disapproving of me—all because of what I have achieved with my weight loss.

In the summer of 2011, I performed at a show and was barely out on the stage before I had the feeling that the audience was not entirely on my ride. I sensed the negative energy coming from the crowd as soon as I walked out.

"Who does she think she is coming out here looking like that?"

"Girl don't look *that* good."

"She must think she's all that now because she lost weight . . ."

"I heard her voice changed when she lost all the weight. I'll bet she can't hold a tune."

I just felt like the audience was standing there thinking these things. I could see their heads shaking, arms crossed, hear their lips smacking. You would have thought they never heard me sing before, let alone know anything about me. I never had an audience treat me like this.

Why were they acting so angry?

I began to sing "I Got This," a song from my second album, as a way to connect with the crowd.

I was doing everything I knew to grab ahold of the audience and take them on the ride, but they wouldn't take my hand. And then it hit me. They no longer saw me as one of them. But you see, to me, I am the same person I've always been. Granted, I might look different on the outside, but I am still that same girl from the

South Side of Chicago who overcame adversity and found a way to do things right by staying positive and finding myself along the way. And yet, I was feeling rejected.

I felt like there were one thousand voices inside my head saying all of the negative comments coming from the audience. There was a point when I wanted to stop singing, stop my show, and say, *"Y'all, it is me. It's still Jennifer."* But I didn't. What was the point? I wasn't going to change anyone's mind that night.

Later that night, some friends who were in attendance told me they were hearing the negative comments from the audience, too. At least I confirmed that what I was feeling was true.

I felt so hurt by this experience. The only thing that made me any different that night was my choice to lose weight and get healthy. I mean, really. Why would anyone rebel against me for that? Was my choice to lose weight somehow touching a nerve for those who think they can't do it?

Folks started using Twitter as a platform for sharing their views about my weight loss. I originally got on Twitter as a way to stay connected to my fans. I wanted to get to know them and give them a chance to know the real me. I don't read every comment that gets posted to my account, but whenever one catches my eye—I'll take the time to address it.

At first, Twitter was an adjustment for me because the people writing had the freedom to say whatever they wanted—good and bad. Naturally, the negative comments are always the ones that get my gander up. I'm a very outspoken woman, and I've spent a lifetime defending myself for one reason or another. My first thought is always to answer back. All of the negative comments started to make me so mad that I stopped checking my account for a while. But I always ended up coming back to Twitter because I liked the interaction with my fans so much, and the positive outweighed the negative.

When it came to discussing my weight loss, people in the Twittersphere had a lot to say. Their Tweets felt more like personal attacks that were rooted in misinformation more than anything else.

Here's a typical Tweet.

*"When you get money that is when you lose weight."*

I wrote back, "My weight loss has nothing to do with money. It's about having the will to do it."

*"My mama said when people get money, they don't need will, they use their money to buy everything."*

My response? "Where there's a will, there's a way."

*"I guess you think you're the shit now because you lost all of the weight."*

Huh? Uh, no.

I wrote back, "I didn't lose weight to impress anyone. I lost the weight so I could be healthy for my son."

———

At the end of the day, I simply couldn't understand how any-one could be mad at me for a goal I set for myself and worked hard to achieve. That isn't about money, fame, or power. It's about will, dedication, commitment, and knowing your self-worth. You can be poor as dirt and have those traits. Money can't buy you val-ues. You just need to know what is important to you and then feel secure in your pursuit to achieve that. The only difference between the haters on Twitter and me is that my will and what I value is what is important to me. Weight loss may not be someone else's goal, but that won't stop me from working toward mine.

The hostile rejection I received was the single biggest hurdle for me to overcome because:


a.  **I didn't expect it, and**
b.  **I didn't know how to handle it.**


I was really upset by this rejection. It reminded me of a friend I had back in high school who told me that he could no longer be my friend because my confidence in myself somehow made him feel like less of a person. I was so hurt that the way I felt about myself made him uncomfortable with who he was.

I decided to speak to Liz in an effort to understand what the rejection to my weight loss was really all about. I figured she might have some firsthand experience in dealing with this type of reaction.

Liz explained that most people see themselves a certain way their entire lives. When they go through a massive change, such as losing weight, they have to learn to see themselves in a new way. It is one of the biggest struggles her members deal with on their journey.

When that gets layered with getting negative energy for doing a positive thing, it oftentimes leads to disastrous results. She told me that she sees this type of reaction in almost every member she works with. They have friends, family members, coworkers, and even mere acquaintances who react in a negative way. She shared that sometimes things get so bad that marriages break up and long-term friendships are lost over this lack of support. I was very relieved to know that what I was feeling and going through wasn't happening just to me. This type of rejection can happen to anyone who is successful in their weight loss, from Jennifer Hudson to Jane Doe.

People get comfortable with the way you are—they have formed their opinion of you based on everything they see and know about you as a person. When you change that up by losing weight, they no longer understand you. Even though you are the same person they've always known, some see you as different. Their perception of who you are has changed based on how you look. Maybe they no longer feel safe, secure, or comfortable with you anymore. Their insecurities get fed by your newfound security with yourself. Liz taught me that when other people reject positive changes you make for yourself, there is always some nerve to get to the root of in those other people. It usually ends up being about fear and lack of self-esteem.

As a way of illustrating just how common this response is, Liz gave me a scenario of four girls who have been best friends since grade school. They went through everything together, including boyfriends, breakups, weddings, babies, and gaining lots of weight. Since they all got heavy together, they supported one another's heaviness. And then one day, one of the girls decided to change her life by taking control of her health and losing the excess weight she'd been carrying around for years. She can't be friends with those people anymore because they can't handle the change. She doesn't want to be around them because everything they do together is centered on eating. They don't exercise, they want to eat out all the time, and they choose all of the wrong foods. Those activities are simply not a part of her life anymore. The rest of the women feel jealous, envious, and angry with her for no longer fitting in with the group. Worse, they are frustrated with themselves because they are still exactly the same. Little by little, they push her out of their circle, until one day they have completely gone their separate ways.

This happens all the time and, as it turns out, is a much bigger problem for women than it is for men. For whatever reason, men don't seem to have as hard a time when one of their buddies loses weight as women do when a girlfriend decides to shed some pounds. Interestingly, men seem to be the majority of the people who come to my rescue on Twitter, often writing, "Why can't you leave her alone?" or "I think what Jennifer has done is terrific. She looks great." And by the way, there are plenty of girls out there who have supported me, too. And to all of you supporters, here's a great big thank-you!

Liz did a great job guiding me through my confusion on this issue by reminding me that I was solid and right in my decision to get healthy. And I was. There was never really a time in my life where this type of rejection would have rocked my world before. No way.

"Would you trade your weight loss for acceptance from others?" Liz asked me.

"Not a chance." I didn't even have to think about my response.

"Would you ever go back to your old weight?"

"Oh, hell no." My answer was that quick.

When Liz framed her questions in that way, it was easy for me to realize that my decision to lose weight was for no one else but me. And when you come from that place, no one—and I mean no one—should have the power or ability to push you back to where you came from.

After giving Liz's questions some thought, I know that, truthfully, I would be willing to gain back weight for a film role, but

only if I had to. Now I know I can control it. I would never care-
lessly go back to my old weight—it would be a choice, a short-term
commitment to gain and then lose that weight. This realization
was big because I really feel like I've got ahold of my eating and
health without any doubt that I would be able to lose the weight
again if I gained. You see, Weight Watchers isn't a diet—it's a commitment to eating for health. Once you've got that, you'll never go
back to your old ways again.

After I discovered the positivity in my new and healthier body,
I began to notice that I wanted to surround myself with other
positive people, too. An organic shift began to take place in my
entire life. If I am going to be a role model who inspires others to
get healthy, then I want to live as the very best example. I didn't
learn how to eat for health until I was a grown woman, but I'm
going to be damned sure my son grows up making the right choices
from the very start. I wish the principles of healthy eating and
exercise were a requirement for kids in school, just like math or
reading. Society puts such an emphasis on being thin and looking
good, but so few people are given the tools early in life to adhere to
these expectations. So when those people walk out into the world,
like I did when I got to Hollywood, it can be a real struggle to
accept that sometimes appearance can be more important than
talent or intelligence. If I had been given the education growing
up, I would have started my journey to health at a much earlier
age. This is why I am so eager to share all of the information

I've been given. I want you to know that there are options out there. If given the right tools, you will be ready and equipped to make your own informed decisions. Where there are options, there is a way. Choices lead to success.

My mama used to tell me that I could do or be anything I wanted as long as I was happy. That was her number one priority for her children. And that is how I want to encourage my son, too. I've seen a glimpse into my son's future—he loves to sing and dance almost as much as he loves to wrestle like his daddy. He is a born performer. He comes to life when he is in front of an audience. Whether it's stealing my spotlight by sneaking out onto the stage and holding his own microphone during a concert in Barbados or insisting he come out with me during an interview on *The View*, my son really knows how to work a crowd. I was exactly like that as a child and now I get to experience what that was like for my mama through my son's eyes. Seeing him shine like that makes me feel so proud. Growing up, I always dreamed of having a sibling I could sing with. Now I get to sing with my son. Munchkin and I sing together all the time, especially when I am putting him to bed at night. He knows his mommy's voice, whether he hears it on the radio, television, or in his bedroom when it's just the two of us together. To the outside world, I'm Jennifer Hudson, singer, actress, and weight-loss ambassador, but to my son, I will always be just Mama. I can't think of a better title!

Becoming a mother is by far my greatest accomplishment. My

son has helped me put everything into perspective and figure out what is really important in my life. Even though I had made up my mind to lose weight before I knew I was pregnant, having my son gave me the best reason not to fail. My mama taught me to always see a cup as half full, and I want to teach that positive perspective to my son, too. I want him to know there is a whole world out there beyond the block he grows up on. Even though he'll grow up in a more privileged environment than I did, he'll still face the world having to make his own decisions. All I can hope for is that I'll do my very best to provide him with the right information and guide him by setting the example by how his father and I live so he will make the right choices.

After becoming a mom, I am most proud of my newfound role as an ambassador of health. There have been such great rewards in seeing how the changes I've made in my life have empowered and inspired others to do the same. I know I touch people's hearts when they see me in an emotionally charged role like Effie White or Winnie Mandela, but nothing had empowered me to help change people's lives until I joined forces with Weight Watchers. I let the world in on my progress by allowing them to monitor my journey to health. I never dreamed that my actions would have such a powerful impact, but God did. He is using every part of me to make a difference in people's lives by spreading my message of health any way I can.

I will never forget a letter I received from a fan shortly after

*Dreamgirls* was released. He wrote me to say that he thought God gave me my acting career because I embraced my gift of singing and shared it with others. Every time I enter a new realm in my career, I realize that there is so much more I am supposed to be doing with my life. And that is why this journey has been so rewarding. It isn't that I've lost eighty pounds and kept it off. No, it's *because* of that accomplishment that I can see people come together—whether it has been my family, fans, or the people on the street—and be inspired by something I did to make a positive change in their lives. *That* is the true meaning of feeling good!

# CHAPTER TWELVE

# I GOT THIS

"Jennifer! Over here!"

"Jennifer, can we get a photo?"

"Jennifer, whose dress are you wearing tonight?"

"Jennifer, Jennifer, Jennifer . . ."

Walking the red carpet has taken on a whole new dimension these days. I get to stand next to the skinny supermodel talking about what I am wearing, about my eyelashes, earrings, and even the color of my toenail polish! Years ago, the only thing anyone wanted to talk about was if I felt insecure as a big girl in Hollywood. And now all they want to focus on is how great I look. Any way you slice it, the emphasis is still about my physical appearance instead of my talent. Does it frustrate me? Sure, but I also know it is part of the game we all play, especially in the looks-obsessed world of Hollywood. Just once I wish someone would make it about being healthy instead of being thin. I've always been comfortable with my size, but I haven't always felt healthy like I do now.

Well, allowing myself to be overweight and unhealthy is a habit I've gladly left in my past—I've got more energy, stamina, and drive than I've ever had. When I am singing "Feeling Good" in my Weight Watchers commercials, that's for real. They couldn't have picked a better song to describe where I am on the journey. And if I can do it, anyone can.

And when I say anyone . . . I mean *anyone*.


I was asked to sing at a very small and intimate holiday gathering at the home of Carole Bayer Sager in late 2010. She has collaborated with everyone from Burt Bacharach to Neil Diamond, Marvin Hamlisch, Michael Jackson, Quincy Jones, Michael McDonald, James Ingram, Donald Fagen, Babyface, and even Clint Eastwood. I was a surprise performer that evening in a room full of billionaires, including Barbra Streisand, David Foster, Diane Warren, and *American Idol* executive producer Nigel Lythgoe. Although it wasn't planned that way, it felt as if everyone there had something to do with my career. I had to kill it with the two songs I was there to sing or there could have been disastrous results.

Earlier in the day, producer and composer David Foster had invited me to his beautiful home in Malibu to work on the arrangements for my performance. We spent a couple of hours together and came up with something absolutely amazing. Because of David, I went into the evening with enough confidence to get me through what could have been the most intimidating and terrifying performance of my career.

Before my show began, I was seated next to Barbra Streisand for dinner. I was nervous to sit next to her because she is such a powerful influence on my singing, of course. I had met Barbra earlier in the year at a pre-Grammy party that Clive Davis hosted. Ever since I signed with Clive, he has asked me to perform at the parties he gives. Clive's gatherings are events more than they are parties. He always makes me feel so special by including me in the evening. For this particular pre-Grammy show, Clive asked me to sing two Barbra Streisand songs: "People" and "The Way We Were."

"And, Jennifer," he said, "Barbra is going to be there."

Now hold up.

He was asking me to sing two of Barbra Streisand's biggest songs . . . for Barbra Streisand? I knew that both songs were challenging for even the best singers, so I was terrified. To make matters worse, he gave me this task with less than seventy-two hours to prepare. But when Clive asks, you don't question; you just do it. I had no choice but to do what I always do—rise to the challenge and learn those songs cold.

So when I sat next to Barbra the night of Carole's Christmas party, I was hoping she had liked the pre-Grammy performance.

Things could have gotten pretty awkward if she didn't. From the moment I sat down, Barbra and I began chatting like we were long-lost best friends. She said she was fascinated by my experiences with Weight Watchers and asked me to tell her all about it.

Seriously.

I began talking with such ease as I told her how simple the plan is.

"I don't think I could ever do that because I need to have my pasta," she said.

I just smiled because that's how I felt, too, before I started Weight Watchers.

"You can eat pasta. You can eat anything you want as long as you stay within your Points," I responded back.

In that moment, we were just two girls talking about weight. I have no idea if she ever gave the program a try, but I know I did my best to lead her toward that choice.

Barbra and I were still talking when Carole came by the table to ask me if I minded that Babyface sang first.

"He said he doesn't want to follow Jennifer Hudson . . ."

We both laughed and I happily obliged her request. Babyface was amazing and would have been just as good whether he followed me or not that night. And then it was my turn to sing. As I did my rendition of "O Holy Night," I looked into the small crowd and felt like I was singing in a dream. I was thrilled to be there but extremely relieved when I was done so I could relax and enjoy the rest of the night.

Toward the end of the evening, Nigel Lythgoe came over to say hello. Nigel hadn't seen me since I lost my weight. His jaw was on the floor as I stood in front of him looking like a brand-new woman.

"I had no idea . . . ," he kept saying over and over to me as he shook his head in total disbelief.

I wanted to say, "I could have always changed this." But in that moment, we both acknowledged that my weight was no longer an issue.

So many people miss out on true talent because they can't get past a look. At the end of the day, losing weight was easy, but finding talent? Now that's hard. I didn't say what I wanted to that night, but I think Nigel knew exactly what I was thinking. I just smiled and said good night.

As the old saying goes, *success is the best revenge.*

It's not that I really had a need to get revenge on anyone—I just wanted to be a breakout example of how no one should be judged on or limited by their looks. Appearance can always be changed, but the talent stays the same. I don't regret all of the things I missed out on by not being given certain opportunities, because my path has led me to who I am today. And for all of that, I am made extremely proud and grateful by the people I meet on the street, in elevators, on airplanes, and everywhere else I go, who tell me that I have inspired them to make a change in their lives. There is nothing that gives me a greater sense of fulfillment than knowing that how I am living my life has a positive impact on so many others. Being a role model comes with a great responsibility, but one I will gladly take on if it means getting other people to the same place that I am. And inspiring others is where I find my inspiration to carry on this lifelong and life-changing important message of health. That is the greatest reward.

In February 2011, I received a call to appear on the final season of *The Oprah Winfrey Show*. I had been a guest several times before, but this visit would be the most poignant because it would be my last, as Oprah's show was ending. My schedule was as busy as it had ever been. I don't drink, smoke, take drugs, or party. Working is my vice. I have a tendency to spread myself a little thin because I hate to say no, especially to someone like Oprah.

When her staff called to book the show, I had already committed to an event in Dallas for Jerry Jones, the owner of the Dallas Cowboys, which Jamie Foxx had called and asked me to do as a personal favor to him. Although there had been some talk about a blizzard in Chicago that week, I thought I could fly to Dallas, do the show, and make it back with enough time to do Oprah's taping the following day. The snowstorm, dubbed by the press as "the blizzard of the century" came and went two days before I flew to Dallas. By all standards, I thought it was a safe bet to go.

I went to Oprah's studio for a rehearsal and sound check on Thursday morning. As soon as I was done, I caught a private plane to Texas, where I was met by a helicopter that was waiting to whisk me off to the venue. Everything was falling perfectly into place.

I did the show, thinking it was all good—that is until I saw my tour manager giving me the signal to wrap things up early. He was mouthing the words, "It's snowing."

Snowing?

In Chicago?

No . . .

In Texas!

That hadn't happened for years.

The weather had gotten so bad that the private plane I had flown in on would not be able to take off. We sat on the plane for an hour before the pilot came out of the cockpit to break the news to us. Apparently, we would not be going anywhere that night. I wanted to tell the pilot to just fly the damn plane, but I remembered something my mama used to say: "Without your life, you can't do anything." And she was right.

Oprah would understand—right? *Right?* I was trying to convince myself of that for the rest of the night. I was supposed to be back in Chicago by five a.m. Friday morning and I was still sitting in Texas trying to figure out how to make that happen.

"Can we take a train?" I asked. But there were none that would get me there on time.

"How about driving to the next city where it isn't snowing so I can catch a flight back from there?" I was getting desperate.

One thing was for sure. We couldn't just sit there waiting for it to stop snowing.

Finally, my tour manager found a commercial flight from Dallas–Fort Worth International Airport that was taking off within the hour, but we still had to drive through the snowstorm to get there if we were going to make it.

Somehow, we were able to get to the airport with enough time to go through security and board the flight. The only seats they had left were the last row in coach. I didn't care. They could have put me in the baggage hold if it meant getting back in time to do the show. As luck would have it, I was on the cover of the in-flight magazine that month, so as I made my way to the back of the plane, I could see every single person look at their copy of the magazine, then look at me and say, "It's her."

"Yup. It's me, all right. How ya doin'?" I was trying my best to find the humor in the situation. I was fine, too, until I heard the pilot announce that this flight was going to be delayed.

Unfortunately, the lines of communication kept getting mixed up. Oprah's producers were being given different stories about why I was late. So Oprah was hearing a whole bunch of different things from her team. I have found that you get a lot further saying things the way they are instead of trying to hide the facts. Eventually, the truth comes out, so what's the point of trying to cover it up? I had been adamant about being honest with Oprah's team. "You will not lie to Oprah!" I was very clear in my intention.

These types of situations get frustrating because issues get created that could have otherwise been avoided. If her producers knew the reality of our situation, I am sure they would have done whatever they could to work around it.

We finally arrived in Chicago late Friday morning, which meant we were already delayed several hours for the taping. My manager arranged to have my hair and makeup people waiting in a car at the airport so I would be camera-ready when we got to Oprah's studio. They did the best they could given the bumps and turns along the way.

When we arrived at the studio, I rushed to my dressing room to finish getting ready. About fifteen minutes later, I looked in the mirror to find Mama O standing behind me.

I swear, you could hear ominous soap opera music in my head, like something dramatic and bad was about to happen.

"Umm, what happened?" she rightfully and respectfully asked.

I told her the truth. I explained that I had been to Dallas to do a show for Jamie Foxx and Jerry Jones. I thought we would make it back in plenty of time until it started to snow in Texas. Oprah was incredibly kind and understanding. She said she knew something had to be wrong because I had never missed a commitment and I am almost always on time. She told me that all I had to do was let her team know what was really happening so they could make arrangements on their end. She was upset with my team for not being candid. I completely understood and respected where she was coming from.

"Jennifer, you have all the power you need, but it is up to you to decide what you're going to do with it." She spoke to me like a loving and caring mother.

I listened to what she was saying very closely because I knew she was talking from experience. I learned a valuable lesson that day, and I told her so.

Oprah was right. You see, we *all* have the power to choose how we are going to handle every situation we are faced with throughout our lives. We are in control of the decision we make whether it's about work, relationships, parenting, or our health.

No matter what I have done in my life, whether singing, acting, or becoming a role model for taking control of my health and wellbeing, it all comes from an extremely authentic place. I wrote this book because I want you to have a sense of who I am, where I've come from, and what I've been through so you know my journey has been totally real.

God blessed me in so many ways, but I don't think my true calling was to be famous or to make a lot of money. I feel like God put me on this path to be a positive influence by helping others find their true selves. If I can't make a difference in someone's day, then all of my fame means nothing because if I am not serving God's purpose, then all of this will have been in vain. Our culture is obsessed with three things—fame, fortune, and appearance. I dreamed about being famous, about making my dreams come true, and about being thin. I've been on both sides of all of those things.

I've struggled. I've been an unknown trying to make it. I've been overweight. I could easily live without the fame and the fortune— but the one thing I could never give up is how healthy I feel now that I've lost what was weighing me down.

The most important things to me on this earth are God, my family, and, last but certainly not least, my health. I can't really imagine living without any of them. There have been many times throughout my life when both my faith and will have been tested. That's just life. I've always been able to push on and persevere when even the darkest of clouds hung over my head. God gave us free will, which means we all have the option to make the right choices in our lives. I've never cared whether the majority of people agree with what I believe because if I don't believe in something, I can't get behind it. But if I do, you can be sure that it's the real deal.

For me, gaining control of my health was a long-term struggle that, for many years, I didn't even realize I had been battling. Now that I've got it under control, I realize that I wasn't living in the way God intended for me. But you know what? I'm okay with that because without all of those experiences, there's no way I could fully appreciate everything that I now have as a result of losing weight and living healthy. It would be insanely greedy to ask for more. I'm grateful for everything that's happened along the way. All I want is to be healthy and happy so I can be around to sing and act for decades to come.

So, here we are—at the end of our journey together. Isn't it time to believe in yourself enough that you are willing to take chances in your life like the ones I've taken in mine? What about loving yourself enough to give it everything you've got and make the commitment to get rid of the things that have been weighing *you* down? Will you finally give yourself permission to break free from the chains that have bound you or will you stay exactly where you are, thinking it's fine? Look, if you don't like what you see in the mirror, don't break the mirror. If you're tired of being on that diet roller coaster and are finally ready to get off that ride forever, you have the power, the choice, and now the tools to make that happen. Life isn't about what cards you are dealt—it's about how you play that hand. Take it from me. I truly know.

I want to wish you my love, support, and inspiration in your journey. Remember, you're making a lifetime commitment to health. It won't happen overnight, but if you stick with it, I promise, it will come to pass.

In Good Health,

# ACKNOWLEDGMENTS

To my family. You are amazing and my reason for being.

To my JHud team, including Allison Azoff Statter, Stefanie Tate, Damien Smith, Lisa Kasteler, Samantha Hill, Marla Farrell, Graehme Morphy, Teri Martin, Matt Johnson, David Lande, Jamie Young, and the incomparable Walter Williams III. Thank you for not limiting me and allowing me to be who I am and for supporting my every dream and effort to continue to grow. That gift is what makes you all such a great team!

To my editor, Carrie Thornton, and everyone at Dutton for allowing me this fantastic opportunity to spread my wings and for giving me the chance to share my story through my own words. Thank you to Brian Tart, Christine Ball, Amanda Walker, Stephanie Hitchcock, Monica Benalcazar, Carrie Swetonic, and the entire Penguin team for your support and guidance to get my message out there. Also, thank you to Mel Berger, my literary agent, who helped take this vision to a reality.

Thank you to Weight Watchers, Weight Watchers, Weight

Watchers! There is not a day that goes by that I don't say Weight Watchers is the greatest thing ever created! It really is! And I want the world to know it. To Liz Josefsberg, David Kirchhoff, Cheryl Callan, Donna Fontana, Danielle Korn, Veronica Bertran, Joyce King Thomas, Kathy Love, Sharon Ehrlich, and Danny Rodriquez—I love you guys!

Now, I had to save my family and fans for last because you have lived with me, you have watched me live, and through it all y'all have stayed next to me. I love you all so much for that! I'm so proud of all of my family, friends, and fans who have decided to make a life change, too. You amaze me.

Finally, without God nothing would be possible.

Weight Watchers Online offers members thousands of recipes and helpful tips. I've included some of my favorite Weight Watchers recipes for you to enjoy.

# Weight Watchers Recipes

## Main Meals

## Desserts

# ★ MAIN MEALS

# Tex-Mex Scrambled Eggs

Course: Breakfast
*PointsPlus*® Value: 4
Servings: 2
Preparation Time: 18 min
Cooking Time: 10 min
Level of Difficulty: Easy

Jalapeño and cumin give these scrambled eggs a bit of heat. They're topped with a homemade spicy salsa for even more flavor.

## Ingredients
14½ oz canned diced tomatoes, fire-roasted variety
¼ tsp chili powder, chipotle variety
2 Tbsp scallions, green part only, minced
2 Tbsp cilantro, fresh, minced
1 Tbsp fresh lime juice
¼ tsp table salt
⅛ tsp black pepper
2 large eggs
3 large egg whites
¼ tsp dried oregano
¼ tsp table salt
⅛ tsp black pepper
⅛ tsp ground cumin
1 spray cooking spray
2 small shallots, minced
1 medium jalapeño pepper, seeded, minced (don't touch seeds with bare hands)

## Instructions
To prepare salsa, pour tomatoes into a fine-mesh strainer set in sink; press on tomatoes to drain off all liquid, leaving about 1 cup of diced tomato. Spoon tomatoes into a medium bowl; stir in chili powder, scallion, cilantro, lime juice, salt, and pepper. Stir salsa; set aside while making scrambled eggs.

To make eggs, in a medium bowl, beat together eggs, egg whites, oregano, salt, pepper, and cumin; set aside.

Coat a medium nonstick skillet with cooking spray; heat over medium heat for 30 seconds. Add shallots and jalapeño; cook, stirring occasionally, until shallots are tender, about 3 minutes. Pour egg mixture into skillet; cook until eggs are almost cooked through, scrambling occasionally, about 4 to 5 minutes. Serve eggs topped with salsa or salsa on the side. Yields about 1 cup of eggs and ½ cup of salsa per serving.

## Notes

If you can find canned tomatoes with chipotle chiles, use them and omit the chili powder in the salsa. You can also save time by using your favorite spicy jarred salsa instead of making your own.

To make this recipe truly Tex-Mex, top with some baked tortilla strips (could affect *PointsPlus®* values).

# Bacon, Egg, and Hash Brown Stacks

..................................................

Course: Breakfast
*PointsPlus®* Value: 4
Servings: 4
Preparation Time: 8 min
Cooking Time: 14 min
Level of Difficulty: Easy

This is a nice twist on the usual potato-and-egg breakfast. Leave an extra "stack" in the refrigerator for a quick, microwave-reheatable meal.

## Ingredients

2 sprays cooking spray
4 frozen hash brown potato patties, prepared without fat
2 large eggs
3 large egg whites
3 oz Canadian-style bacon, finely chopped
1 Tbsp scallions, minced, green part only
⅛ tsp hot pepper sauce, optional
⅛ tsp table salt, or to taste
⅛ tsp black pepper, or to taste
8 tsp ketchup, hot and spicy variety (optional)

## Instructions

Coat a large nonstick skillet with cooking spray. Place hash brown patties in skillet; cook over medium heat on first side until golden brown, about 7 to 9 minutes. Flip patties; cook until golden brown on second side, about 5 minutes more.

Meanwhile, coat a second large nonstick skillet with cooking spray; heat over medium-low heat. In a large bowl, beat together eggs, egg whites, bacon, scallions, hot pepper sauce, salt, and pepper; pour into prepared skillet and then increase heat to medium. Let eggs partially set and then scramble using a spatula. When eggs are set, but slightly glossy, remove from heat; cover to keep warm until hash browns are finished cooking.

To assemble stacks, place 1 hash brown patty on each of 4 plates. Top each with ¼ of egg mixture and serve with 2 teaspoons of ketchup. Season to taste with salt and pepper, if desired. Yields 1 stack per serving.

## Notes

Finely diced turkey bacon makes a nice alternative to the Canadian bacon in this recipe. Just make sure to cook the bacon before adding it to the eggs (could affect *PointsPlus*® values).

# Italian Pepper and Egg Sandwiches

Course: Sandwiches
*PointsPlus®* Value: 5
Servings: 4
Preparation Time: 10 min
Cooking Time: 12 min
Level of Difficulty: Easy

This comfort-food sandwich is great for breakfast, lunch, or dinner. It's made with a lot of pantry staples, perfect anytime you need a quick meal.

## Ingredients

    2 tsp olive oil
    1 small onion, thinly sliced
    1 large green pepper, such as a cubanelle, thinly sliced
    1 tsp minced garlic
    4 large eggs
    3 large egg whites
    ½ tsp table salt, or to taste
    ¼ tsp black pepper, freshly ground, or to taste
    4 reduced-calorie hamburger rolls, toasted if desired

## Instructions

Heat oil in a large nonstick skillet over medium heat. Add onion and pepper; sauté until tender and light golden, about 7 to 9 minutes. Add garlic; cook, stirring, until fragrant, about 30 seconds. Set vegetables aside.

In a medium bowl, beat together eggs, egg whites, salt, and pepper. Scramble in same skillet over medium heat until almost cooked, about 1 to 1½ minutes. Add vegetables back to skillet and gently mix; continue scrambling until eggs are set but not dry, about 30 seconds to 1 minute more.

Top each roll bottom with about ¾ cup egg mixture; cover with roll tops and serve. Yields 1 sandwich per serving.

# Tropical Chicken Salad
# with Orange Vinaigrette

Course: Main meals
*PointsPlus*® Value: 7
Servings: 2
Preparation Time: 18 min
Cooking Time: 0 min
Level of Difficulty: Easy

Tropical fruit and cucumber make this main dish salad super-refreshing. The next time you're grilling chicken breasts*, make extra for this recipe.

## Ingredients
  2 Tbsp orange juice
  1 Tbsp rice wine vinegar
  2 tsp olive oil
  ¼ tsp table salt
  ¼ tsp black pepper, freshly ground
  4 cups mixed baby greens
  5 oz chicken breast, stewed, without skin
  ¾ cup pineapple, fresh, cut into chunks
  ¾ cup mango, fresh, cut into chunks
  ¾ cup cucumber, seedless, cut into chunks
  ¼ cup mint leaves, fresh, cut into thin strips
  ¼ cup red onion, thinly sliced

## Instructions
  In a large bowl, stir together orange juice, vinegar, oil, salt, and pepper until blended.

  Add salad greens, chicken, pineapple, mango, cucumber, mint, and onion; toss to mix and coat. Serve immediately. Yields about 3 cups per serving.

## Notes
  *You can buy precooked chicken strips if you prefer.

  Give this salad a Cuban spin by adding a sprinkle of cumin to the dressing and swapping out the mint for fresh cilantro.

# Chicken and Cheese Quesadillas

Course: Main meals
*PointsPlus®* Value: 9
Servings: 4
Preparation Time: 12 min
Cooking Time: 10 min
Level of Difficulty: Easy

A Mexican classic with endless variations: Try Monterey Jack cheese and jalapeños, pico de gallo, and black beans or shredded jicama and mango salsa.

## Ingredients

- 2 cups (chopped) chicken breast without skin, roasted, chopped, or shredded
- 1 tsp fresh lime juice, or to taste
- ¼ tsp Durkee ground cumin, or other brand
- ¼ tsp table salt
- 8 medium whole wheat tortillas, about 6 inches each
- ½ cup fat-free black bean dip, spicy variety
- 6 Tbsp low-fat shredded cheddar cheese, sharp variety
- 2 medium scallions, green part only, diced
- 4 sprays cooking spray
- ½ cup salsa
- 2 Tbsp reduced-fat sour cream

## Instructions

In a small bowl, combine chicken, lime juice, cumin, and salt; toss well to combine.

Place 4 tortillas on a flat surface and spread each one with 2 tablespoons of bean dip. Top each with about ⅓ cup of chicken and then sprinkle each with 1 tablespoon of cheese; divide scallions over top. Cover with remaining tortillas and gently press down on each one.

Coat a very large nonstick skillet with cooking spray; place over medium heat. Cook quesadillas in a single layer until golden brown on bottom, about 2 minutes. Flip quesadillas and press down on them with a spatula; cook until golden brown on second side, about 2 to 3 minutes more. Remove to a serving plate and cover to keep warm (or place in oven); repeat with remaining quesadillas.

Slice each quesadilla into 4 pieces; serve with salsa and sour cream. Yields 1 quesadilla, 2 tablespoons of salsa, and 1 teaspoon of sour cream per serving.

## Notes

For even greater flavor, look for a low-fat seasoned Mexican cheese blend.

If you want to make the chicken from scratch, marinate it in a mixture of lime juice, cumin, and chipotle chili powder for 30 minutes before grilling or pan-frying (with cooking spray); then shred with a fork.

# Feta-Stuffed
# Chicken Burgers

Course: Main meals
*PointsPlus®* Value: 7
Servings: 4
Preparation Time: 15 min
Cooking Time: 16 min
Level of Difficulty: Easy

Olives, roasted peppers, and feta add great flavor to these burgers. Complete your meal with our light Greek Salad.

## Ingredients
- 1 pound uncooked extra-lean ground chicken breast
- 1 Tbsp fresh oregano
- ¼ tsp garlic powder
- 7 Tbsp feta cheese, crumbled
- 4 items reduced-calorie hamburger rolls
- 1 cup lettuce, romaine, cut into thick strips
- ⅔ cup roasted red peppers, sliced (without oil)
- 5 small olives, black, sliced (about 4 tsp)

## Instructions
Preheat grill or broiler.

In a medium bowl, combine chicken, oregano, garlic powder, and feta; divide mixture into four balls and then press them gently into patties.

Grill or broil patties until internal temperature of burgers reaches 165°F, about 7 to 8 minutes per side.

Serve each burger on a bun with ¼ of lettuce, ¼ of peppers, and 1 teaspoon of olives. Yields 1 burger per serving.

# Grilled Yellowfin Tuna with Teriyaki Sauce

..........................................................................

Course: Main meals
*PointsPlus*® Value: 5
Servings: 4
Preparation Time: 8 min
Cooking Time: 9 min
Level of Difficulty: Easy

A summertime pleaser. The teriyaki sauce is simple to make and so full of flavor: rich, tangy, and thick.

## Ingredients

1 spray cooking spray
3 cloves (medium) garlic, finely minced
2 Tbsp ginger root, fresh, finely minced
1 Tbsp sherry cooking wine, or mirin
½ cup low-sodium soy sauce
½ cup orange juice
¼ cup water
3 Tbsp packed brown sugar, dark variety
1 Tbsp cornstarch
16 oz yellowfin tuna, 1-inch thick

## Instructions

Coat grill rack with cooking spray; preheat grill to high.

To make teriyaki sauce, in a small saucepan, combine garlic, ginger, sherry, soy sauce, orange juice, water, sugar, and cornstarch. Boil for 5 minutes, stirring constantly, until thick.

Coat all sides of tuna with teriyaki sauce. Grill, flipping once, brushing on more teriyaki sauce as fish cooks, about 4 minutes for rare, or longer to desired degree of doneness.* Serve with arugula tossed with your favorite salad dressing, or some oil, vinegar, salt, and pepper (could affect *PointsPlus*® values). Yields about 3 ounces of tuna per serving.

## Notes

*Grill 3 minutes per side for a 2-inch tuna steak cooked to rare. Or cook longer until desired degree of doneness.

You can also broil the tuna. Just preheat the broiler, along with the pan, to high.

# Spicy Beef Tacos

• • • • • • • • • • • • • • • • • • • • • • • • • • • • • • • • • • • • • • • • • • • • • • • • • • • • • • • • • • • • • •

Course: Main meals
*PointsPlus®* Value: 7
Servings: 4
Preparation Time: 12 min
Cooking Time: 13 min
Level of Difficulty: Easy

You get two tasty tacos in a serving. Add your own touch with fresh chopped cilantro, scallions, or tomatoes.

## Ingredients
    3 sprays cooking spray, divided
    2 cloves (medium) garlic, minced
    ¾ pounds uncooked lean ground beef (with 7% fat)
    1½ tsp Durkee ground cumin, or other brand
    1½ tsp ground coriander
    ¾ tsp table salt, or to taste
    1½ cups canned diced tomatoes, with jalapeños or green chilies
    8 small corn tortillas, lightly toasted just before serving if desired*
    2 cups lettuce, shredded
    ½ cup low-fat shredded cheddar cheese, sharp variety
    ⅓ cup salsa

## Instructions
    Coat a large skillet with cooking spray; heat over medium-high heat. Add garlic; cook, stirring, until fragrant, about 30 seconds to 1 minute. Add beef; cook until browned, breaking up meat as it cooks, about 5 to 6 minutes. Add cumin, coriander, salt, and diced tomatoes; cook, stirring occasionally, until liquid is almost absorbed, about 5 to 6 minutes.
    Place tortillas on a flat surface. Top each with about ¼ cup beef, ¼ cup lettuce, 1 tablespoon cheese, and 2 teaspoons salsa. Fold tortillas in half and serve. Yields 2 tacos per serving.

## Notes
    *To toast tortillas, coat a baking sheet with cooking spray. Place tortillas on top and coat with cooking spray. Heat in a 300°F oven until slightly crisp but not too crisp that they break when folded.

# Shrimp with Zucchini and Tomatoes

Course: Main meals
*PointsPlus*® Value: 4
Servings: 4
Preparation Time: 8 min
Cooking Time: 10 min
Level of Difficulty: Easy

Keep a bag of large frozen shrimp on hand for this quick and easy sautéed meal. The juices from the tomatoes add a wonderful flavor to the sauce.

## Ingredients

- 1 Tbsp olive oil, extra-virgin, divided
- 1 medium zucchini, cut into ¼-inch slices
- 1 pound shrimp, large-size, peeled, and deveined
- 1 cup grape tomatoes, cut in half
- ½ tsp dried oregano
- ½ tsp table salt
- ¼ tsp black pepper, freshly ground, or to taste
- 1½ tsp minced garlic
- ¼ cup water

## Instructions

Heat 2 teaspoons oil in a large nonstick skillet over medium-high heat. Add zucchini in a single layer; increase heat to high and cook until bottoms are golden, about 2 minutes. Flip zucchini and cook until golden on other side, about 2 minutes more. Using a slotted spoon, remove zucchini to a plate.

Heat remaining teaspoon oil in same skillet. Add shrimp; sauté 1 to 2 minutes. Add tomatoes, oregano, salt, and pepper; sauté until shrimp are almost just cooked through, about 1 minute. Stir in garlic and water; sauté, stirring to loosen bits from bottom of pan, until shrimp are cooked through and tomatoes are softened, about 1 to 2 minutes more. Return zucchini to skillet; toss and serve. Yields about 1¼ cups per serving.

## Notes

Try this with fresh basil instead of, or in addition to, the oregano (just stir it in right at the end).

Grate some lemon zest over top and/or sprinkle with fresh lemon juice, if desired.

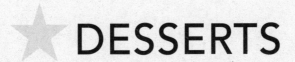 DESSERTS

# Frozen Mud Pie Sandwiches

Course: Desserts
*PointsPlus*® Value: 3
Servings: 10
Preparation Time: 15 min
Cooking Time: 0 min
Level of Difficulty: Easy

Low-fat coffee frozen yogurt gives this childhood favorite a grown-up taste.

### Ingredients
20 chocolate wafers, or vanilla wafers
1¼ cups low-fat coffee-flavored frozen yogurt, softened
10 tsp fat-free fudge topping

### Instructions
Spread 2 tablespoons of frozen yogurt on top of each of 10 wafers.

Drizzle 1 teaspoon of fudge topping over each yogurt-covered wafer. Cover with remaining wafers and gently press together to make sandwiches. Wrap each mud pie in plastic wrap and freeze for 1 hour. Yields 1 per serving.

# Cookies and Cream
# Freezer Cake

Course: Cakes
*PointsPlus®* Value: 5
Servings: 12
Preparation Time: 12 min
Cooking Time: 0 min
Level of Difficulty: Easy

Our lightened-up version of icebox cake is a summer crowd-pleaser. It'll hit the spot on hot, humid days.

## Ingredients

- 3½ oz ready-to-eat vanilla pudding, about 1 cup
- 3 cups Cool Whip Whipped Topping Lite, aerosol, or similar product
- 9 oz Nabisco Famous Chocolate Wafers, or similar product (should be about 3 inches in diameter each)
- 1 oz bittersweet chocolate, shavings

## Instructions

Line bottom and sides of a 13- to 14-inch-long pan with plastic wrap, making sure you use a big enough piece so that you have enough extra wrap to cover prepared cake.

In a medium bowl, gently fold pudding into whipped topping.

Take a wafer and spread about 1½ tablespoons of cream mixture over cookie surface. Top with another wafer and spread about 1½ tablespoons of cream mixture over second cookie; repeat to form a stack of about 6 cookies and cream. Carefully turn stack on its side and place in pan so cookies are standing on their sides. Repeat with remaining cookies until you create 1 long row of cookies and cream in pan. (Reserve any broken cookies to crumble over top as a garnish.)

When cake assembly is complete, use a spatula to scoop up any cream that has oozed out of sides of cookies and place back on top of cake.

Wrap plastic tightly around cake in pan and freeze immediately for a minimum of 2 hours.

Slice cake on a diagonal into 12 pieces and sprinkle each piece with shaved chocolate. Yields 1 slice per serving.

## Notes

Feel free to swap chocolate pudding for the vanilla, if desired.

# Mini Chocolate-Chip Cookies

Course: Desserts
*PointsPlus*® Value: 1
Servings: 48
Preparation Time: 10 min
Cooking Time: 6 min
Level of Difficulty: Easy

Go ahead and grab a few of these bite-size cookies. They might be little, but they pack a big chocolate punch.

## Ingredients
2 Tbsp butter, softened
2 tsp canola oil
½ cup packed brown sugar, dark variety
1 tsp vanilla extract
⅛ tsp table salt
1 large egg white
¾ cup all-purpose flour
¼ tsp baking soda
3 oz semisweet chocolate chips, about ½ cup

## Instructions
Preheat oven to 375°F.

In a medium bowl, cream together butter, oil, and sugar. Add vanilla, salt, and egg white; mix thoroughly to combine.

In a small bowl, mix together flour and baking soda; stir into batter. Add chocolate chips to batter; stir to distribute evenly throughout.

Drop 48 half-teaspoons of dough onto one or two large nonstick baking sheets, leaving a small amount of space between each cookie. Bake cookies until golden around edges, about 4 to 6 minutes; cool on a wire rack. Yields 1 cookie per serving.

## Notes
Indulge your craving for an intense chocolate experience. Buy a 3-ounce bar of fine chocolate with a percentage of 75 or higher on the

label. The percentage indicates the combined amount of cocoa bean and added cocoa butter in the chocolate. The higher the percentage, the greater the chocolate taste and the less sweet the product. Chop up the bar and use it instead of the chocolate chips (could affect *PointsPlus*® values).

# ABOUT THE AUTHOR

**Jennifer Hudson** is a Grammy-winning international pop star and Academy Award–winning actress. She is the current spokesperson for Weight Watchers.

CONNECT ONLINE
www.jenniferhudson.com
facebook.com/jenniferhudson
twitter.com/IAmJHud

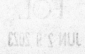